VALENTIA LIFEBOATS

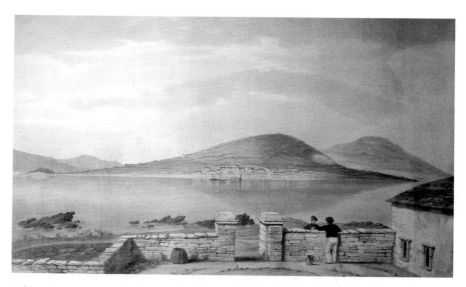

Lifeboat Station at Renard Point. Photo: courtesy of Valentia Island Heritage Centre.

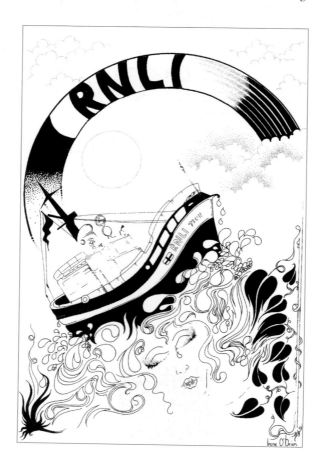

VALENTIA LIFEBOATS

A HISTORY

DICK ROBINSON

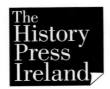

The
History
Press
Ireland

To Tess, my wife, soul mate and best friend. To Richard and Tina, our son and daughter for their patience, tolerance and encouragement I can but say thank you. Thanks to two wonderful grandsons Jack and Caoimhin. From his perch in front of the TV Jack would call out, 'Come on Granda, "Lifeboat Luke" is on.' Caoimhin just smiles and no more is needed – he too can melt the heart.

In the South-western Islands of Ireland the people
have a blood-creed all their own.
Kinship is important to them to an unlimited degree.
In the islands they nurse each other's children, marry each
others kindred and bury each other's dead.
Valentia is the most beautiful of all the islands.
I know, because I have wept for the beauty of it
amongst the many things that make South-western Islanders weep.
Such as the laying down of Loved Ones in Kilmore Graveyard,
where the grey headstones glisten on the hill that drowns the encircling bay.

Liam Mac Gabhann

First published 2011

The History Press Ireland
119 Lower Baggot Street
Dublin 2
Ireland
www.thehistorypress.ie

© Dick Robinson, 2011

The right of Dick Robinson to be identified as the Author
of this work has been asserted in accordance with the
Copyrights, Designs and Patents Act 1988.

British Library Cataloguing in Publication Data.
A catalogue record for this book is available from the British Library.

ISBN 978 1 84588 707 0

Typesetting and origination by The History Press
Printed in Great Britain
Manufacturing managed by Jellyfish Print Solutions Ltd

CONTENTS

ACKNOWLEDGEMENTS

Caherciveen Library Staff

Commissioners of Irish Lights

Connaughton Marcus RTE and *Seascapes* producer/presenter

Cooke, Liz, editor of *The Lifeboat* and her editorial team

Curtin, Brendan, Valentia and Irish Naval Service

Curtin Pat, Valentia

Denton, Tony, Lifeboat Enthusiasts' Society (LBES) honorary treasurer

Duffy, Joe RTE, on-scene presenter of *The Gay Byrne Show* from Valentia Lifeboat
  Station

Egan, Michael and Bridie

Falvey John, Valentia Radio O/C

Farr, Mrs Elsie, Portishead

Foran, Richard, lifeboat operations manager, Valentia

Francis, John G., honorary secretary, LBES

Gallagher, Paddy, late honorary secretary, Valentia lifeboat

Greene, Raphael (RIP), Coachford and Valentia

Griffin, Kathleen of Irish Coastguard Administration

Houlihan, Joseph (retired mechanic) and his wife Kathleen

Houlihan, Leo, mechanic at Valentia Lifeboat Station

Kerry County Library Archivist and Archives at Tralee

Kipling, Ray, former deputy director of the RNLI

Lavelle, Des, Valentia

Leach, Nicholas, LBES, honorary photographic records officer

Mackey, Adrian of Valentia

Mc Sweeney Tom, former RTE Marine Correspondent and *Seascapes* presenter

Millman, Anne of the RNLI Poole

Morris, Jeff, LBES honorary archivist

Murphy, Mr Eamonn, Valentia

Murphy, Paudie of Roche's Point and Valentia

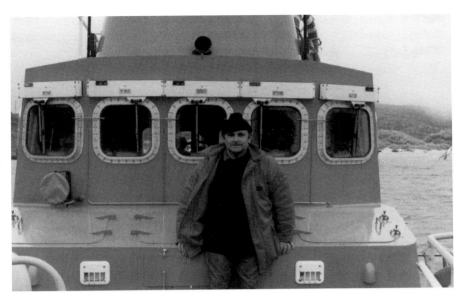

The author on board the Valentia Lifeboat at Derrynane harbour on Sunday 26 July 1987.

Murphy, Seanie, retired coxswain, Valentia

O'Driscoll, Maurice, Valentia and Dublin

Quigley, Richard, coxswain Valentia lifeboat

RNLI Rescue Records Department at Poole

RNLI Dublin Office Airside Swords. Anna Classan, Niamh Stephenson, Eilish
  Matthews

Robinson, Paul, Cobh and Valentia

Sugrue, Brendan, former Valentia Radio O/C

Sullivan, Gene former Valentia Radio O/C

The Gay Byrne Radio Show and Gay Byrne (recovery of scrapbooks and live
  broadcast from Valentia Lifeboat Station)

The History Press for publishing this book and Ronan Colgan and Beth Amphlett
  for their advice and assistance

The Walsh Family – Dermot (coxswain) Carmel Aidan and John. Valentia

Those who appear on the list of Valentia lifeboat crew in a separate list. In my
  youth they fanned the flame of interest in the Valentia lifeboat and the broader
  RNLI

Torpey, Eamon of the Irish Coastguard

Valentia Heritage Centre

Woolhouse, Peter, LBES and Chatham Historical Lifeboat Group

INTRODUCTION

The maroons burst through the January gloom. Knightstown came to life as men, women and children left their Christmas fires and rushed to the lifeboat house. It was 26 December 1946.

'What's wrong?'
'Who is it?'
'Is it a shipwreck?'

There were questions and babble and running feet. The lifeboat station had opened on Valentia only five weeks before on 20 November 1946. Down the cobbled unlit road men, women, and children ran, walked, and stumbled. I remember it. My mother was practically dragging me along as she hurried to the 'back of the watch house' where the old lifeboat shed stood. This was excitement with a capital 'E'. I clutched the tin boat that Santa had recently brought and was carried along with the crowd. Rounding the corner, eyes blinked at the blast of electric light provided by the thumping generator. The whole seaside village's population had turned out. The shiny yellow of the oilskins disappeared into the darkness as the boarding boat left the beach. Soon deck and navigation lights came on and the eighty horse-power Weburn engine roared to life. Chains clanked and the mooring chain was slipped and the buoy dropped overboard. The green starboard light disappeared and the port red light came to view as the C&S lifeboat turned clear of the mooring chains and white water spewed into a wash as she headed towards the Lighthouse at Cromwell's Point, the harbour mouth, and the Atlantic Ocean. A Spanish trawler had been reported in distress off Keownglass Point.

Nobody moved until the boat had disappeared into the Atlantic. Lights vanished and the engine sound faded as the quiet crowd dispersed in twos and threes.

My mother never went to the lifeboat station again. I believe she had seen enough. When the maroons exploded she would kneel on a stool which my father had made at woodwork class in the parish hall. Facing the window which

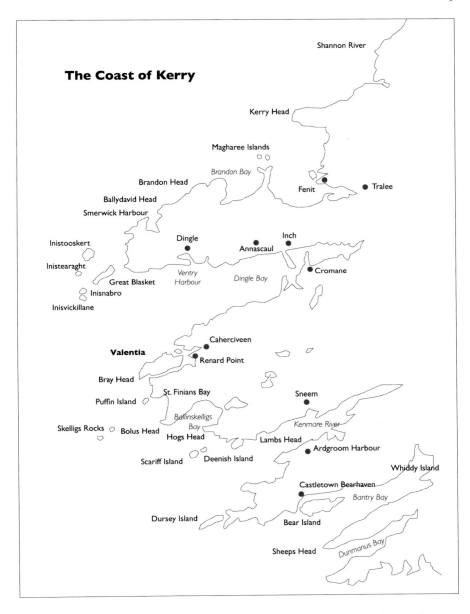

The Coast of Kerry

Shannon River

Kerry Head

Magharee Islands

Brandon Bay

Brandon Head

Fenit ● Tralee

Ballydavid Head

Smerwick Harbour

Inistooskert

Dingle   Inch

Annascaul

Inistearaght

Ventry Harbour   *Dingle Bay*

Great Blasket

Cromane

Inisnabro

Inisvickillane

Caherciveen

Valentia

Renard Point

Bray Head

St. Finians Bay

Sneem

Puffin Island

Ballinskelligs Bay

Kenmare River

Skelligs Rocks   Bolus Head

Hogs Head   Lambs Head

Ardgroom Harbour

Scariff Island   Deenish Island

Whiddy Island

Castletown Bearhaven

Bantry Bay

Dursey Island

Bear Island

Sheeps Head   *Dunmanus Bay*

itself faced the direction of the lifeboat station, she would take her well worn rosary beads, cross herself and help the lifeboat crew in the way she thought best. Because the lifeboats crews are our neighbours or neighbours' children they should never be taken for granted, locally or elsewhere. Where else in society will volunteers, fully aware of all the risks involved take a lifejacket and step into the boarding boat to go into harm's way to save a neighbour or a complete stranger?

For some sixty years now I have been fascinated by those people. I have been privileged to serve in a small way on Valentia lifeboat crew. I am privileged to number the lifeboat people of Valentia amongst my special friends. Through branch activity and the Lifeboat Enthusiasts' Society I am fortunate to be in contact with lifeboat people in many places. Patrick Howarth, in acknowledging the society, wrote the following poem.

The Silent People

There are silent people who rescue others,
From shipwreck and flood and fire,
And vocal people who tell mankind,
What it should and should not desire.
Those who work with the silent people,
Know that always and nevertheless,
Attention turns to the vocal people,
The political and economic people,
The projected and personally purposeful people,
Except when there's sudden distress.

In presenting to the best of my ability the story of Valentia lifeboats I want to honour not only my friends at home on the island of my soul, but all who go to sea in the full knowledge that they may drown, but they must go as somebody is out there. This is for the silent people everywhere …

Note:
Valentia lifeboat has been on swinging moorings since 1946. Some 716 odd times she has put to sea to assist others. The procedure leading to 'the lifeboat slipped moorings' or the 'lifeboat set out' as appears in the text is as follows:

There is a cause of service. Emergency Services are made aware. Honorary secretary is contacted and authorises launch. He or the Shore Attendant at the Station fires maroons (two supercharged fireworks). Volunteer crew get to the station as fast as possible. They get information about the casualty, collect their gear, launch the boarding boat and row to the lifeboat. Engines are started. Rudder was lowered from stowage to at sea position. Boarding boat bowline is secured to moorings. Mooring chain to disconnected and dropped overboard. Lifeboat goes astern to clear the chains before engaging 'Full ahead both engines'.

Since 1980s the crew are summoned by bleeper rather than by maroon. The boarding boat is now a motor one and the steering is no longed clipped up for storage while at the moorings. On some occasions the launching procedure had been done in less than five minutes, in most less than fifteen.

ONE

THE *ORANMORE*

'Valentia lifeboat, Valentia lifeboat, are you reading me please. Over.'

The normal calm had left the voice of the operator at Valentia Radio Station, 'My God, I've lost contact with the lifeboat, I can't raise her.' The radio operator had good reason to be concerned. He, like all coastal dwellers, was only too aware that within the previous twelve months two lifeboats had been lost off the Scottish coast.

The *Longhope*, Orkney's lifeboat had been lost with her crew of eight, while on service to the Liberian ship *Irene* on the 17 March 1969. A loss of contact with Wick Radio had been the first harbinger of disaster. The lifeboat was found upside down at 1.40 p.m. on 18 March. There were no survivors. Lieutenant Commander Brian Miles was then Inspector of Lifeboats in Scotland.

He remembered the occasion when he spoke, as Director of the RNLI, to the Lifeboat Enthusiasts' Society in London on 18 January 1998. He visited each crew member's house personally to bring them the tragic news. Each family asked the question as to what had happened the crew of the *Irene*. All were delighted with the news that they had been saved. Each widow said, 'My husband would have been pleased to know that'. Just a month before now, the operator at Valentia knew, the Frazerburgh lifeboat, on service to a Spanish Fishing Vessel *Opal*, had been overturned, bow over stern, by a giant wave. Five of her six crew had perished. Word went around the coast that Valentia lifeboat was missing. At Kilronan, the Aran Islands lifeboat was launched. Lighthouses and Coast Lifesaving stations were alerted. In Kilrush, as elsewhere, the maroon roared skywards and burst over the town. The marine community rushed to their assembly point. The rest of the town wondered at the noise.

Valentia lifeboat was battling her way through mountains of green sea off Sybil Point, *en route* to assist the motor vessel *Oranmore*, which was in grave difficulties off the mouth of the Shannon. On board the wildly heaving *Rowland Watts* on 20 February 1970 a radio malfunction was the problem. Dermot Walsh, the forty-six-year-old quiet-spoken coxswain was braced behind the wheel. Mechanic

Joseph Houlihan could hear messages on the radio but could not transmit. They were only too aware of what was running through the minds of those ashore. There was no way to let them know that all was well. On altering course to the north-east from Sybil Point, a report from the *Oranmore* to Valentia Radio that she had a target on the radar at that position was intercepted by Joseph Houlihan. Parachute flares were fired and reported. Many Valentia hearts began to beat again.

Valentia lifeboat had earlier been alerted by Valentia Radio Station when the Limerick Steamship Company Vessel *Oranmore* got into difficulties with her engines broken down 9 miles north-north-west of Brandon Head. The lifeboat crew – Coxswain Dermot Walsh, Mechanic Joseph Houlihan, his assistant Patrick Murphy, Bowman Anthony O'Connor, and crew members John Curran, John Curtin and Nealie Murphy set out at 6.05 p.m. on the forty-two-mile passage through the Atlantic storm along the vicious Kerry Coast to the casualty. For five dreadful hours the lifeboat battled through the worst the Atlantic could throw at her and finally arrived off the casualty at 11.15 p.m. For the next two hours the lifeboat stood by while the engineers on the *Oranmore* worked frantically to try and repair the engines. At 1.15 a.m. Captain J.B. O'Sullivan gave the signal that he wanted some of the crew taken off.

With his whole world pitching violently, Dermot Walsh nudged the twenty-eight ton lifeboat forward. Rising between 20 and 30 feet on each giant wave, the ever-present danger was that the seaman on the rope ladder over the starboard side of the *Oranmore* would be crushed between the two boats or that the ship, straining desperately at the hawser of her one remaining anchor, would crash on the foredeck of the lifeboat, crushing the waiting lifeboat men. Years of experience counted. Walsh got it right first time and one man was snatched to safety from the ladder. On the second run in, two more men were snatched from the ladder, but it was impossible to hold the lifeboat alongside for more than a few seconds at a time. Having observed the difficulty of the rescue, Captain O'Sullivan gave the order to abandon ship.

Like all the Barnett class lifeboats, the *Rowland Watts* was sluggish in her response to the helm at slow speeds. Watching the motion of the casualty and reading the seas, Dermot Walsh again coaxed her forward and alongside, but this time a nylon heaving line was secured on board the *Oranmore*. By skilful use of the helm and engines, and with consummate seamanship he brought the lifeboat alongside the ship's ladder as she was being swept aft by heavy seas. This exercise was repeated several times. Sometimes a man successfully jumped and was caught, on other occasions he was grabbed from the ladder. Unfortunately the seventh man, the ship's mate, Joseph Lennon, miscalculated his jump and fell into the sea. Momentarily leaving the scene the lifeboat coxswain grabbed the man with a boat hook and with other crew members managed to haul him over the stern. Mouth-to-mouth resuscitation was immediately applied by the coxswain, followed by mechanic Houlihan, and continued by other survivors, but unfortunately the man was not revived.

The rescue work continued, despite the violent seas, and the remainder of the *Oranmore*s' crew was taken off by 2.10 a.m., when the lifeboat slipped her head rope. As the engines worked astern the port propeller became fouled by a rope, but efforts to force this failed. With ten extra people and one body on board, one engine out of action and no radio transmitter Coxswain Walsh decided to run for Kilrush. The lifeboat arrived at 6.16 a.m. on 21 February in company with the local pilot boat which had guided the lifeboat to the pier at Cappa. Here the lifeboat was met by Garda Superintendent Frank Dooris who gave hot drinks to the lifeboat crew and the rescued men. The Glynn family looked after the lifeboat crew in their home and provided beds at the Riverside Hotel for most of the survivors. Anthony O'Brien, a Kilrush native, went to his home.

At an inquest in Kilrush Dr Kathleen Ryan who had examined the body at the pier, told the coroner, Dr Christopher F. Coughlan, that in her opinion Joseph Lennon died of cardiac arrest due to shock and asphyxia from sudden immersion in the water.

Captain O'Sullivan told the inquest that the last voyage of the *Oranmore* was from Rotterdam to Antwerp where they loaded slag and returned to Limerick.

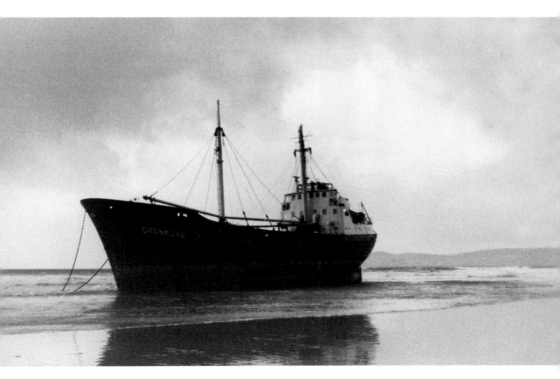

February 1970: The *Oranmore* blown ashore at Banna Strand after her crew had been dramatically rescued by Valentia Lifeboat. She was successfully refloated and returned to service. Photo: Dick Robinson Collection.

They unloaded some of the cargo there and took the balance to Galway. They left for Liverpool at 4 a.m. on 18 February. Because of the storm he had sheltered near Scattery Island for twenty-four hours. On the 19 February he put to sea but again had to return for shelter near Labasheeda. On the 20 February they put to sea at 9.50 a.m. but as they proceeded the weather worsened. Nine miles north-west of Brandon Head the engines stopped. The Chief Engineer informed him that the repairs could not be carried out at sea. A ship called the *Selectivity* came to their aid but attempts to tow the *Oranmore* failed. He then gave the details of the rescue. The coroner, the foreman of the jury, Michael Flynn and Captain O'Sullivan called for extra rescue facilities on the west coast. The coroner, the foreman of the jury and Superintendent Dooris, as well as conveying their condolences to the

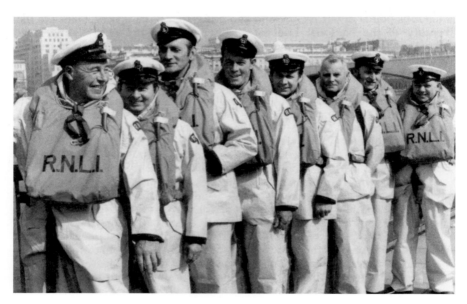

Decorated lifeboatmen in London for the presentation of Gallantry Awards at the Royal Festival Hall on 2 April 1971. From left to right: Second Coxswain Ernest Guy and Motor Mechanic William Burrow both of St Mary's, Scilly Isles, who received a bar to their Bronze Medals (their coxswain, Matt Lethbridge, who received a bar to his silver medal, could not attend). They rescued ten from the Swedish Ship *Nordanahav* on 21 February 1970; Coxswain Dermot Walsh of Valentia, Silver Medal for *Oranmore* rescue; Stephen Whittle for the rescue of three from the trawler *Glenmalure* on the 25 November 1970 (one of those rescued was the then coxswain of Kilmore Quay lifeboat); crew member David Brunton of Dunbar, East Lothian in Scotland who dived overboard from the lifeboat to save a man on 23 December 1970; Pat Houlihan of Valentia, a brother of Joseph, spent some time as mechanic at this station (Bronze Medal); Coxswain Alfred Maddrell of Port Erin, Isle of Man, Bronze Medal for the rescue of two men from the coaster *Moonlight* on 9 September 1970; Coxswain Ronald Hardy of Swanage, Dorset, Bronze Medal for a service to a boy trapped in a cave on 12 September 1970; Coxswain William Harland of Whitby, Yorkshire, Bronze Medal for a service to fishing vessel *Gannet* on 15 July 1970. Photo: courtesy of *The Times*, London.

bereaved family, paid fulsome tributes to the Valentia lifeboat crew. The chairman of the Kilrush Harbour Authority, Jack Fennell, also paid tribute. He pointed out that the authority had voiced their criticism the previous year when the Fenit Lifeboat Station had closed.

Ironically since 1996 County Clare's RNLI station has operated from Cappa, just west of the pier where the *Oranmore* survivors were landed. Kilrush Operates an Atlantic eighty-five class lifeboat *Edith Louise Eastwick*. The station has proved its worth since it opened.

'Man Killed in Storm Drama' headlined the *Evening Press* of 21 February 1970. 'Coast Drama – Man Drowns – 12 Saved' said the *Evening Herald* of the same date. But it was just another day in the life of Valentia lifeboat. At the Royal Festival Hall in London on 21 April 1971 the Silver Medal of the Royal National Lifeboat Institution was presented to Coxswain Dermot Walsh. The rest of the crew were presented with the thanks of the Institution inscribed on vellum for their outstanding performance on the *Oranmore* rescue.

The lifeboat service is not about medals or awards. It is about answering every call for help. It is about dedicated people using their skill and courage. Putting their lives on the line for others, irrespective of race, creed or colour.

TWO

IN THE BEGINNING

The first lifeboat was stationed at Valentia in November of 1864. In a strong editorial on the 3 December 1864, the *Kerry Evening Post* put the case before the people as follows:

The Valentia Lifeboat
One of the most dangerous points of our rock bound and dangerous coast is now, thanks to the liberality of the National Lifeboat Institution, provided with a first class lifeboat of the newest and most improved construction. This boat passed through Tralee on to Caherciveen last week, having been brought from London to this port free of expense by the Limerick and London steamer. The boat is, as we have said, of the very first class as to size and build. She is thirty two feet long, seven feet four inches wide and pulls ten oars double banked. Her self-righting qualities were tested (in the Regents Canal Dock, Limehouse), with the most satisfactory success before she was sent from London. She righted almost instantaneously, and eighteen men, all sitting on her gunwale, would not bring her down; and she has floatage to carry eighty men. The water she shipped was self-ejected, through patent valves, in fifteen seconds.

The following are some of the qualities of the new boat: Great lateral stability – speed against a heavy sea – facility for launching and taking the shore – immediate discharge of any water breaking into her – the important advantage of self-righting if upset – strength – storage room for a number of passengers. The boat was built by Messrs Forrest of Limehouse. The transporting carriage of the boat, which was built by Mr. J. Robinson of Kentish Town, London, was also tried on the occasion and found to answer very well. The whole cost of the lifeboat establishment, amounting to £508, has been presented to the National Lifeboat Institution by a benevolent lady after whom the boat has been named, Mary.

The boat having been landed in Tralee free of expense, the local public are expected to contribute some two hundred pounds to fit up a suitable boat house, and pay thirty pounds a year to organize a crew, etc. The parent

Institution is prepared to pay all rewards etc. that may be allowed to the crew for actual services in saving life etc.

Mr. J. Kearney White, Inspecting Officer of Coastguards at Caherciveen, has been most zealous in rendering the National Institution every assistance in the organization of the lifeboat station and in obtaining contributions in aid of its future support. Mr. White has received contributions and promises as published in our advertising columns, but these do not cover the outlay that Mr. White has already incurred. That gentleman has, on the faith of the liberality of the people of Kerry, built a commodious boathouse, and has made other payments on account of the lifeboat. The outlay has, as we have said, exceeded two hundred pounds. Mr. White and those gentlemen connected with Iveragh who are acting with him in this good work, think this a very opportune moment to press the claims of the Valentia lifeboat upon the county, and we think so too. Therefore do we now call public attention to the matter.

We can not conceive it necessary, particularly after such storms, accompanied by shipping disasters as these islands have just gone through, to urge the claims of the lifeboat upon our readers. We will only remark that we miss very many names which ought to be on the list. Both our County Representatives are absent from the list, as also is the Representative of the Merchants of our Borough. These gentlemen ought to figure amongst the highest subscriptions on the list. We also notice that the mercantile community of Tralee are absent as a body. Two or three gentlemen have subscribed – but only two or three – and we need not remind those among our merchants who trade in ships, that the cause of shipwrecked mariners has the strongest claim upon them. We would remind the public throughout our county, from all sides and all ranks, that this is a cause in which all ought to deem it a privilege to assist.' Mr. Kearney White was indeed a good mentor for the new lifeboat crew. Twice in the same year while serving at Blyth in Northumberland he was awarded Silver Medals for Gallantry by the RNLI.

The first rescue was on 10 February 1852. The sloop *William and Mary* was driven ashore near Blyth in an east-north-easterly gale and her crew took to the rigging. Mr Kearney White put out in a fishing coble and with a crew of six rescued the four men. The crewmen were so weak that they could not haul in a rocket line fired from the shore. Again on 25 October 1852 in an easterly gale, Mr Kearney White put out in the Blyth lifeboat. The Russian barque *Victoria* was the casualty. In difficult conditions the crew of fourteen from the barque were rescued

Trinity College was the first on the list of subscribers, and the first twenty-five names appear in Appendix No. 1.

In the issue of the *RNLI Journal*, dated 1 January 1865, the announcement was more brief:

Valentia – A new lifeboat station has been established by the National Lifeboat
Institution at Reenard Point, on the coast of Kerry, facing the island of Valentia,
and a new 32 feet ten-oared lifeboat, with transporting carriage, has been placed
there. The boat will not only be available for any vessels going ashore off the
entrance to Valentia Harbour, but she can also be transported overland by good
roads to Dingle and Ballinskelligs Bay, north and south of the island. A commodious boathouse has been erected on an eligible site. A benevolent lady, resident
in Berkshire, who had previously given the Institution the cost of a lifeboat for
the North West Coast of England, presented the society with £508 to defray
the whole cost of this lifeboat establishment, the boat being named, at her
request the *Mary*. A free passage was readily given to the lifeboat and carriage as
far as Tralee, by the London and Limerick Steamship Company on board one
of their steamers.

The 'benevolent lady' referred to in the announcement was Miss Mary Wasey of
Newbury. The lifeboat cost £223 6s, the carriage cost £96 4s and the boathouse
at Renard Point, on lands belonging to Trinity College, cost £155. The boat was
built of mahogany.

The first coxswain appointed was William Shanahan and Mr James Kearney
White was appointed as honorary secretary. Because the only reliable crew available was on Valentia Island, the station was moved to the island in 1869. The
Reenard boathouse was demolished and rebuilt on the island at Knightstown, on
a site granted by the Knight of Kerry. The boathouse was subject to a 100-year

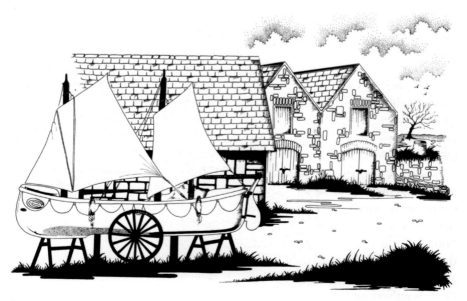

RNLB *Mary* at Valentia.

lease. This was entered on 4 August 1869. The plot for the boathouse measured 50 feet in length, outside the wall, from north to south and 24 feet in width and was bounded on the north by the strand of the seashore, on the east by the Knight of Kerry's boathouse and a portion of strand and on the south and west by a portion of waste ground at the rear of Market Street. The rent was one shilling payable yearly on the 1 November. The lease strictly limited the use of the land for a lifeboat house only. The lease was signed at Portmagee by Peter Fitzgerald, Knight of Kerry, before William Lambert and was signed at 14 John Street, Adelphi, London by Richard Lewis, a Barrister at Law, before W.R. Smith. (Richard Lewis was Secretary of the Institution) Mr Kearney White remained in office until 1866, when he was succeeded as honorary secretary by the Knight of Kerry. The Knight held the office until 1875, when it passed to John O'Driscoll. John O'Driscoll died on 8 November 1888 having served thirteen years as honorary secretary and was succeeded by his son Alexander O'Driscoll. John O'Driscoll, Lloyds Agent and representative of the Shipwrecked Fishermen and Mariners Benevolent Society, was the person who had first requested in 1858 that the Lifeboat Institution station a boat at Valentia. John was chairman of the local committee. On the 13 March 1874 the Second Assistant Inspector reported 'Crew On Exercise, Remarkably Good Oarsmanship'. Of the six service launches that the *Mary* made from Valentia, the only effective one was on 16 February 1875. On that date a boat containing part of the crew of the ship *Sydney Dacres*, bound from San Francisco to Liverpool, arrived at Knightstown on Valentia Island. The *Sydney Dacres* had been abandoned at sea and fourteen of her crew were still missing. The *Mary* was launched immediately. After rowing for seven hours in search of the missing sailors they were found, 'on the South West Skelligs Rock, and landed at Valentia at midnight, after a very hard day's work'. Rewards to the crew totalled £12 10s. In that year some work was done to the boathouse. T. Gulliver was the contractor.

On 3 May 1875 the brig *Carrie Anne* of Plymouth was reported in difficulties off the Skelligs. When the lifeboat arrived her services were declined. Rewards of £6 12s were paid. In 1880 in the month of June the lifeboat was re-named *Crosby Leonard*, when she was appropriated to a legacy of Mr Crosby Leonard of Bristol. Under this name she never launched on service.

Coxswain Shanahan died in early 1888. On the 12 February the Committee of Management voted £10 to his widow. He had served as Coxswain for twenty-two years. On 24 January 1890 a new lifeboat was sent to Valentia. She bore the same name as her predecessor – *Crosby Leonard* – and bore the Official Number 174. She was a 34 foot self-righting lifeboat. Her cost was £352 and the builders were Willams and Robinson of Thames Ditton. A new carriage was also supplied. The lifeboat was brought by train to Killorglin from Cork by the Great Southern and Western Railway. She was rowed from Killorglin to Valentia as the railway line had not proceeded beyond Killorglin at that point in time.

The only fatality at that time associated with Valentia lifeboat occurred on the 7 February 1890. The tragic event actually happened in Killorglin, some 30 miles from Valentia.

The *Kerry Sentinel* of the 12 February 1890 carried the story as follows, 'A poor man named Lenehan was killed last week by the accidental overturning of a cart by which he was crushed to death on the spot'. It was the following entry in the 'London Notes' of the same *Kerry Sentinel* on Saturday 22 February 1890 that related the incident to Valentia lifeboat:

> At a recent meeting of the committee of Management of the Royal National Lifeboat Institution, London, a letter was read from Mr. Alexander O'Driscoll, Justice of the Peace, Valentia detailing the circumstances under which the unfortunate man Thomas Linehan of Killorglin met with a fatal accident while the new lifeboat carriage was leaving for Valentia. The Committee expressed their deepest regret at the sad accident and sent Mr. O'Driscoll, honorary secretary at Valentia a cheque for £100 for the widow of Lenehan who has been left with a large helpless family.

In *The Lifeboat* of 1 May 1891 the following entry appeared: 'Also £100 to the widow and children of a man who was accidentally killed by being run over by a lifeboat carriage at Valentia, Ireland.'

This entry caused some confusion in research. It suggested that the accident actually happened at Valentia. This was clarified by the Kerry newspapers.

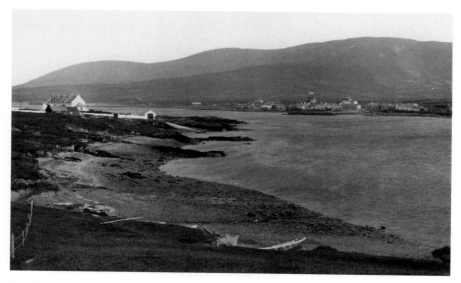

The Portmagee Channel, with Portmagee on the right. The white houses and yard on the left are the coastguard houses. Photo: courtesy of National Library of Ireland.

On the 8 September 1892 the cart track at Carriglea was widened to allow the lifeboat to be brought by road from Knightstown and to allow her access to the water. The new *Crosby Leonard* launched on service only four times from Valentia. There was one effective service. On 13 January 1894 a boat from the barque *Berna*, registered in Dammam, with sixteen men and one woman on board arrived at Valentia. Its captain reported that the *Berna* was in a sinking condition and had lost most of her spars and sails. She was inward bound from Jamaica to Le Havre with a cargo of timber. Due to language difficulties it was unclear as to whether there were other lifeboats adrift or persons remaining on board the distressed ship. The *Crosby Leonard* lifeboat put to sea under the command of Coxswain Frank O'Donoghue. Well used to rowing seine boats, the lifeboat was rowed out into the Atlantic by a willing crew. They contacted the *Berna* near the Bull Rock. Coxswain O'Donoghue put three men – Phil Sullivan, Jeremiah O'Connell and Jim Driscoll – on board. They were to sail as best possible towards Valentia with whatever canvas remained. The lifeboat returned to Valentia to enlist the help of a steamer to tow the crippled vessel to port.

Throughout the night Jeremiah O'Connell remained at the helm, while Phil Sullivan and Jim Driscoll set what little canvas was left intact. Then they proceeded to check the holds and the hull. They returned to O'Connell shaking and shaken as demonic screams came from the for'ard hold. 'Satan has come for us' they concluded as the screaming waxed and waned. By dawn O'Connell could take no more. 'If Satan has come for me I will meet him head on and be done with it.' Armed with a broken spar he went to the hold and ripped the cover off it. Within was a black pig at that time an unknown quantity on the edge of the world in Valentia. Most likely a Eurasian boar, the pig's normal habitat would be Africa. The *Berna* was on passage from Jamaica to Le Havre. Given the large trade and slave trades between Jamaica and Africa the presence of the black pig would be quite normal.

The lifeboat returned with a steamer and the *Berna* was brought to Valentia. A few days later the *Berna* was taken in tow by the tug *Flying Fox* to London. A salvage claim was taken in the Dublin High Court and the sum of £500 was awarded to the lifeboat crew who were – Coxswain Frank O'Donoghue, Phil Sullivan, Jeremiah O'Connell, Jim Driscoll, Paddy Burke, Jamsie Burke, Paddy Lynch, Sonny Shea and Michael Falvey. No record seems to exist of the fate of the black pig. Perhaps given the distress he caused the lifeboat men when he arrived at Valentia his goose was cooked.

During a period of thirty years there had been little rescue activity by the Valentia lifeboat. Of ten service launches only two were effective and the results were fourteen people landed and one ship saved. At a meeting of the Institution's Committee of Management in London on 14 November 1895 it was decided to close the lifeboat station and the lifeboat was withdrawn. The first boat was sold to the Burke family and ended her days as a cattle boat. The second lifeboat was broken up in 1896.

An Extract from the Minutes Book of the RNLI on 21 February 1896 reads as follows:

Portmagee (Co. Kerry) Mr C.G. O'Connell of Portmagee, called attention to the desirability of forming a lifeboat station at this place, which is at the West End of Valentia Harbour. He asserted that it was a great mistake ever to place a lifeboat at Knightstown, at the east end of Valentia Harbour (Known as Valentia, which station has just been discontinued) as it was too far inland and no proper crew could be obtained there, whilst Portmagee was in every way suitable for a Lifeboat Station. An Excellent crew could, he stated, always be obtained at this place.

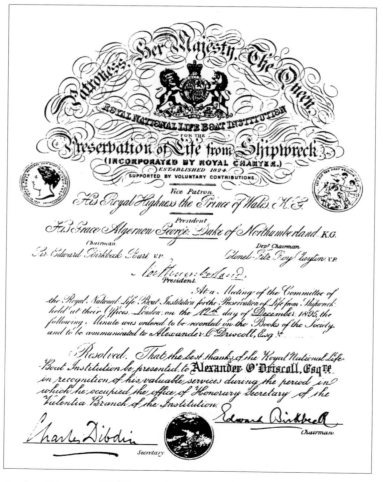

A copy of the vote of thanks given to Alexander O'Driscoll for service as honorary secretary, 12 December 1895. Photo: courtesy of Mrs Mary Sheedy (*née* O'Driscoll).

On 12 March: Committee decided that Mr O'Connell be thanked and informed that the Committee, having given this matter most careful consideration, could see no reason to alter their decision to withdraw the Lifeboat from the locality.

It would be remiss, however, to suggest that the lifeboat men at Valentia did not have their fair share of adventure. In August of 1864 two test lifeboats were sent to Valentia. *The Times* of London on 10 December 1864 carried a letter from Richard Mahony JP of Dromore, under a most accurate heading of:

Extraordinary Lifeboat Adventure
Sir,
A description of a strange lifeboat adventure during the late gales may be of interest to many of your readers.

In August last, two whale boats constructed on the principles of the life-boat arrived in the harbour of Valentia, on the South West Coast of Ireland. They were consigned to the charge of Mr. Kearney White, inspecting officer of Coastguards in the District, and were intended to be subjected to certain experimental trials which would test their qualities in all circumstances.

No weather occurred sufficiently heavy for such experiments until the late November gales. Some most successful trials then took place in the heavy Atlantic seas off this Western coast, and the behaviour of the boats was most satisfactory.

They differ slightly in construction. In the one built by Mr. Forrest of Limehouse, the property of self-righting in case of being overturned is most prominent. This quality does not exist to the same degree in the other boat built by Mr. White of Cowes, which is a much lighter craft, but her steadfastness and irreversibility, as will be seen, are most extraordinary.

The 26th November last (1864) opened on the West Coast of Ireland with a heavy gale from the west-north-west. The barometer had gone down to 28.90. The force of the wind was 10. A tremendous sea was running and breaking wildly on the headlands of Dingle Bay. In one place it was observed from some miles off bursting over a cliff more than one hundred feet high.

Everything was considered suitable for a thorough trial of the lifeboats. Both were accordingly got ready for the occasion. They were merely five oared Whale boats provided with airtight compartments and clearing valves for discharging the water.

Mr. Forrest's boat was manned by the coxswain and half the local crew, who are at present in training for a large national lifeboat just presented to this station by an English lady. The other boat was manned by the Coastguard Crew and steered by the inspecting officer himself. Both crews were provided with Captain Wards lifebelts. Within the harbour all was comparatively smooth, vessels riding easy to their anchors, but the Gale was so strong that the boats made headway with great difficulty, the wind sometimes driving the oars out of the rowlocks up over the men's heads in spite of the utmost efforts to keep them down. Slow progress was made thus towards a passage leading out into a wild bay called Lough Kay, which lies outside the harbour of Valentia to the north. Here the seas were running mountains high and it became evident that no boat of any description could live long under it. Mr White, however, still being determined to try the boats even under these circumstances, made his final arrangements for a bold experiment. He directed the boat which accompanied him to lie in comparative shelter under Lamb Island (a small grassy island 78 feet high, over which the seas were making full breach) so that she might watch the fate of her consort and render assistance if possible. Then with his own Coastguard crew (In White of Cowes boat) he dashed out into the bay, watching each tremendous roller and rounding her to meet it. About a quarter of an hour passed in this struggle when a great tidal wave was observed by spectators gathering itself about a mile to seaward. Distinguishable by onlookers far inland like a mighty Andes towering over lesser mountains, this Atlantic Giant swept in, extending right across the bay and leaping far up the cliffs on their side. In the opinion of experienced seamen who observed it, this sea would have swept the decks of the Great Eastern like a raft. As it neared the devoted boat its appearance became more terrific. The water shoaled there from ten to seven fathoms and changing its shape with the conformation of the ground below, that which had been a rolling mountain rose into a rushing cliff of water.

Never were six men in more desperate circumstances, yet what men could do was done boldly and steadily. The rule laid down for meeting a desperate sea is to pull against it with the utmost speed; but for meeting such a sea as this no rule was ever made. Cheering his men forward, the steersman put his boat right at it, calculating nicely to meet the sea at a right angle. Steadily, as if spurting in a race, the men strained at their oars and gliding on an even keel, like an arrow the boat entered the roaring avalanche, its breast towering twenty five feet above her and overhanging.

The Inspecting Officer was steering and the chief boatman who was pulling the stroke oar were hurled headlong over the boat's stern by the falling sea. Had she not been of extraordinary strength, owing to her particular double sided construction, she must have shivered like a band box. Crushing her bodily fathoms down, the sea bore her astern at lightening speed, tearing away her rudder irons and steering crutch by the pressure. The steersman was caught head downwards as she passed, by some projecting hook or spur of a rowlock and dragged thus for a few seconds; then he found himself suddenly freed and rising rapidly. On reaching the surface he met the chief boatman, already afloat, but looking very much confused. The latter afterwards described himself as being conscious of receiving some tremendous impetus which caused him as he imagined, to turn a series of somersaults under water. Though cased in very heavy waterproof boots, thick pea jacket and oilcloth covers, the lifebelts supported them with perfect ease.

The sea which has hurled them overboard had beaten the rest of the crew down as they bent over their oars in a stooping posture, each man on the thwart before him. The bowman alone was stunned, the remaining three retained perfect consciousness; they had their eyes open, but all around was total darkness. They describe their sensation as like being whirled in an express train through a railway tunnel, but whether they were in the boat or in the sea they could not distinguish at the time. At length a faint dawn of light reached their eyes, increasing rapidly, and they were conscious of rising through the green water, and at last they emerged through the broken foam sitting each man in his place.

The first thing that their eyes met as they rose to the surface was the buoy of the Kay Rock close alongside them. The buoy is by measurement over four hundred yards from the place where the sea had first struck their boat. She had been shot about a quarter of a mile under water and had risen in the exact position where she had entered the sea. A spare rowlock and a pair of boots were lying loose in the bottom of the boat giving clear evidence that she had not once turned over during her extraordinary submarine passage. The oars had all been lost but one, and with this the men had managed to keep her head to the seas, though she was drifting fast upon the rocks astern.

In the meantime the crew of the other boat watched the whole occurrence, but so appalled were these hardy fishermen by the appearance of the sea and by the sight which they had witnessed that they refused at first to pull out to the rescue in the face of what appeared to be certain death. The brave man who commanded her however, Edward O'Neill, was determined to save his comrades or share their fate. By dint of entreaty and command he got them to pull into the bay, skilfully watching his time, some times putting his boat away from the rolling breakers. Sometimes driving her over the seas shipping seas forward and on both sides. He succeeded in picking up the officer and the chief boatman, after they had been nearly half an hour in the water. Then they pulled away for the other boat and reached her as she was drifting on the rocky shore over which the sea was breaking furiously. A very few minutes later and the boat and men would have been pounded to fragments on the sharp ledges which were rising black at intervals through the foaming water. They supplied the drifting boat with oars which they had picked up from the water and both crews worked their way back into the harbour without loss of life or even the slightest injury.

The time during which the boat remained submerged is difficult to arrive at. Under such circumstances seconds seem like minutes both to the actors and the spectators, but as far as I can judge from pretty fair data, she must have been two minutes under water.

I can scarcely expect anyone who reads this statement of so wonderful a preservation from destruction to believe it. I could not believe it myself at first. Nor
could any, save those who witnessed it.

I will only say that anyone who takes the trouble to investigate the particulars
as I have done, by close examination of both the actors in the scene and the
spectators, will be convinced that I have understated the circumstances.

I am, Sir, Your Obedient Servant,

Richard Mahony JP Dromore, County Kerry.

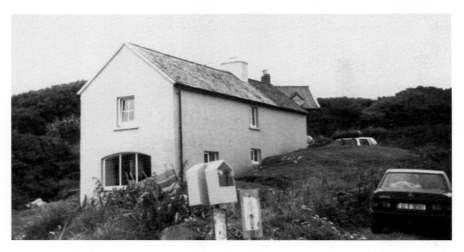

Former Derrynane Lifeboat House. Derrynane Lifeboat Station was opened from 1844 to
1855. The boat never launched on service. Photo: Dick Robinson.

Reading the letter practically a century and a half later the incident still seems fan-
tastic. One thing is certain, that Richard Mahony JP was very well versed in things
maritime of his day. The *Great Eastern* launched in 1858 by Isambard Kingdom
Brunel had a designated tonnage of 18,914 and was soon to lay the Atlantic Cable
from Valentia to Newfoundland. The largest ships of the day were a mere 5,000
tons. The Beaufort Scale (see Appendix 2) was in its infancy as Sir Francis Beaufort
had died in 1857. Captain Wards lifebelts had been completed in 1861, being tested
at Whitby in Yorkshire when the lifeboat there capsized. Henry Freeman, the only
crew member with one of Ward's lifebelts, was the sole survivor. He became coxswain of the lifeboat there and saved 300 lives in that capacity. On the basis that the
letter was based on an investigation by a Justice of the Peace who was also a marine
expert, his claim to have under-rated the case is totally credible.

On whatever grounds the Committee of Management based their decision to
close the station in 1895, the quality of the seamanship certainly left nothing to
be desired at Valentia.

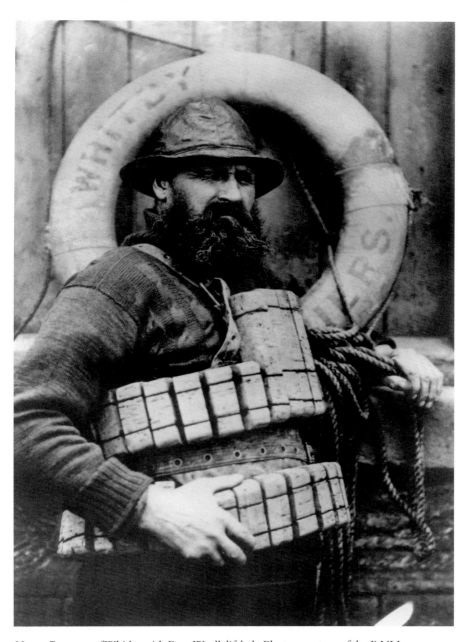

Henry Freeman of Whitby with Ross Ward's lifebelt. Photo: courtesy of the RNLI.

THREE

THE INTERIM YEARS

Lifeboat Development

By the time another lifeboat would be stationed at Valentia, design and development of lifeboats would have come a long way. In fact, research had been going on since the late eighteenth century. Following the death of the Bishop of Durham Nathaniel Crewe, a trust in his name was set up to address the problem of shipwreck. In 1786, the trust asked Lionel Lukin, a London coach builder and inventor, to apply his method of making vessels unsinkable to one of their local cobles. This consisted of the use of cork and watertight buoyancy chambers. The resulting vessel operated successfully at Bamburgh, Northumberland for several years.

In March 1789, the ship *Adventure* was wrecked in the mouth of the Tyne. Hundreds watched helplessly from the shore as the sailors dropped to certain death. No assistance could be rendered to them because no suitable boat was available. Following this appalling tragedy a group of local businessmen formed the consortium which was called 'The Gentlemen of Lawe House'. The 'Gentlemen' offered a prize of two guineas for a suitable model lifeboat. The designers Henry Greathead and William Wouldhave entered models. In adjudicating the designs, the Gentlemen decided that since neither design was totally satisfactory that they should split the prize. Wouldhave stormed from the meeting in disgust. Greathead was then commissioned to build a lifeboat. His finished product, *The Original*, incorporated many of Wouldhave's ideas, and became the prototype for another thirty lifeboats built over a period of fourteen years. Eighteen were stationed in England, five in Scotland and eight were sent abroad. Greathead was voted £1,200 by Parliament and fifty guineas by the Society of the Arts; nevertheless, near the maritime museum in South Shields stands a memorial which acknowledges both Henry Greathead and William Wouldhave as inventors of the lifeboat.

The National Institution for the preservation of lives and property from Shipwreck (Now the Royal National Lifeboat Institution) was proposed by Sir William Hillary. The meeting founding the Institution took place at the City of London Tavern on 4 March 1824. The site of the City of London Tavern is now occupied by the Brown Shipley Building in Bishopsgate London E.C.3. It is between Gracechurch Street and Threadneedle Street. A plaque on the wall of that building states:

> On this site where formerly stood the City of London Tavern, the Royal National Lifeboat Institution was founded as a voluntary body at a meeting held on the 4th March 1824, presided over by the Archbishop of Canterbury, Dr. Charles Manners Sutton.

The pulling and sailing type of lifeboats like the *Crosby Leonard* boats carried a massive amount of gear. Masts, spars, oars and ropes, even when stowed away, made 'going forward' a daunting task, comparable with an assault course. The massive amount of rope and cordage had to be constantly monitored by the coxswain and the District Inspector to ensure that they were reliable and serviceable when needed. The sails were of canvas, made from the finest flax and tanned with bark to render them rot-proof. The sheets and halyards were made of yacht manilla and the standing riggings made of steel wire. The rig was a standing fore lug jib and standing mizen lug sail. This prevented the use of a tiller, so steering was by means of an oar or tiller ropes, whichever the coxswain found most convenient. The amount of canvas carried was small in comparison to the fishing fleets and the sails were effectively storm sails. Drop keels were fitted and could be lifted to facilitate coming about or running before the wind. In the event of the keel, which was made of iron, being damaged by wreckage or rocks, it could be jettisoned by pulling out the retaining pin.

Each boat was equipped with a drogue or sea anchor. This is a canvas bag, conical in shape, which was towed astern in following seas. Storm oil was also carried. The oil can would be punctured with a marlin spine and oakum – a cordlike substance used to caulk or seal the seams between the timbers of boats – plugged into the hole to regulate the flow of the oil, so that it seeped slowly and calmed waters near the wreck. It was also towed over the bow of the boat in heavy seas so that the oils would drift astern and prevent the seas from breaking. Various types of oil were tried, including colza, linseed, fish seal and paraffin, but there was no significant difference.

Oars were the subject of considerable research. Oars breaking during launching or beaching operations could prove fatal. In 1866, trials were carried out. They were extensive and involved thirty-eight different types of wood. Different species of ash and fir were used, including Quebec Yellow, American Red, Oregon Pine and Baltic White. Oars were found to be the best when made from young trees in Norwegian and Baltic woods, followed by oars made from planks of the same wood. Oregon Pine was also good. A balance had to be struck between oars which would break under ordinary conditions and ones which would not break if the lifeboat struck bottom in shallow waters and thereby capsize her. Later oars were balanced with lead inside. White oars were to be used on the starboard side and blue oars to port. The official, and not a little condescending, RNLI. circular on the subject stated, 'The orthodox terms, starboard and port, are rarely used in lifeboat work since many lifeboatmen are unaccustomed to nautical phraseology'! The crew of the Penlee lifeboat, operating from Newlyn, immediately reversed the placings of the oars as a gesture of protest against the tone of that particular instruction.

Lifeboat development continued slowly, but the sea continued to kill. In December 1886 searing storms savaged the north west coast of England. The German barque *Mexico* was outward bound from Liverpool to Quayaquil in Ecuador with general cargo. She had a crew of twelve. When she was wrecked in the Ribble Estuary, the lifeboat *Laura Janet* under the command of Coxswain William Johnson and with a crew of twelve was launched from St Anne's in Lancashire but was found upturned at Airdale the next morning. All thirteen volunteer lifeboatmen were killed. Lytham lifeboat had in the meantime rescued the twelve Germans, returning to sea to search for St. Anne's lifeboat, it found that the Southport lifeboat, which had also launched to the *Mexico*, had capsized, drowning all but two of her crew. Twenty-seven men in all perished in the disaster and left sixteen widows and fifty orphans.

Following this disaster, the operational outcome was that every boat in the fleet was surveyed and allotted a number. This has become the Official Number allotted to each boat by the RNLI (ON 1218 is the *John and Margaret Doig* based at Valentia). In 1887, Mr George Lennox Watson was appointed as consulting naval architect to the RNLI. In 1890 he designed two new lifeboats, one for sailing and one for pulling. Neither was self-righting. The sailing boat was 43 feet long with a beam of 12 feet and 8 inches and weighed 11 tons. This made her difficult to launch from a beach but once at sea she was excellent. The pulling boat was 38 feet by 9 feet and 4 inches, was also admirable at sea and difficult to launch from a beach.

In 1897, Watson told a House of Commons inquiry into the RNLI. 'With the large sailing boats, I think we can get a better boat by abandoning the self-righting principle, but I would not risk it with the smaller boats'. The financial outcome was that Sir Charles Macara, a Scotsman, who had made a fortune from cotton and lived in St Anne's, took up the cause of the RNLI. He carefully planned his campaign and on 1 October 1891 launched what was titled, 'The world's first ever street collection for charity'. The lifeboat flag day is still a cornerstone of fundraising.

Watson also addressed the problem of building a steam lifeboat, as powered lifeboats seemed to be the solution. Indeed Sir William Hillary, the founder of the RNLI, had proposals for a steam lifeboat, but these proposals were never acted on.

The first steam lifeboat, *Duke of Northumberland*, was completed in 1890. She was 50 feet in length, had a beam of 14 feet 3 inches and a depth of 3 feet 6 inches. Of steel construction, she had fifteen watertight compartments and 72,000 rivets were used in the construction. Not self-righting, it was stated that, 'her stability vanishes at one hundred and ten degrees, i.e. when her mast is as far below the water as to make an angle of twenty degrees with the surface.'

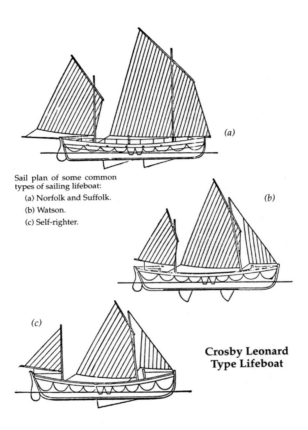

Sail plan of some common
types of sailing lifeboat:
(a) Norfolk and Suffolk.
(b) Watson.
(c) Self-righter.

**Crosby Leonard
Type Lifeboat**

The boat required a technical crew of four – a chief engineer, an assistant engineer and two firemen. She could get up steam in twenty-five minutes from cold, or in fifteen minutes if the boiler had been heated. She was driven by a form of jet propulsion, as propeller propulsion was seen as impractical. In all, six steam lifeboats were built and propeller or screw propulsion was rendered possible in later versions by enclosing the propeller in a tunnel. On studying all the various launching methods, coastal peculiarities, and the overall area of cover it was obvious that steam lifeboats would never provide a powered craft for general use and that another alternative would have to be sought, as she had to lie afloat and could not be shore launched. That rescue by oar and sail would be the norm for a long time to come was accepted. It was decided to look at the petrol engine and the practicality of fitting it to the existing boats as a means of

THE 'WATSON' PULLING AND SAILING LIFE-BOAT

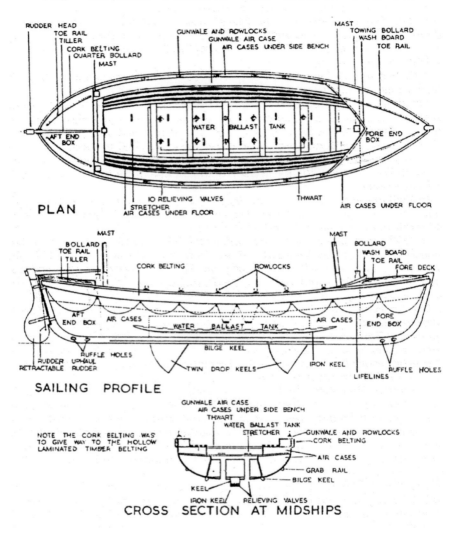

PLAN

SAILING PROFILE

CROSS SECTION AT MIDSHIPS

secondary power. A rather awesome list required that a petrol engine for use in lifeboats be:

- Inside a water-tight casing that would be unaffected by seas breaking inboard.
- The casing could not be airtight, as a supply of air had to reach the carburettor.
- The engine would have to be as near automatic as possible.
- Lubrication must be self renewing.
- Power output had to be steady and unaffected by the motion of the boat, even if she was virtually standing on end.

S R [SELF RIGHTING] TYPE LIFE-BOAT

THIS TYPE WAS TO BECOME THE MAINSTAY OF THE FLEET FOR MANY YEARS

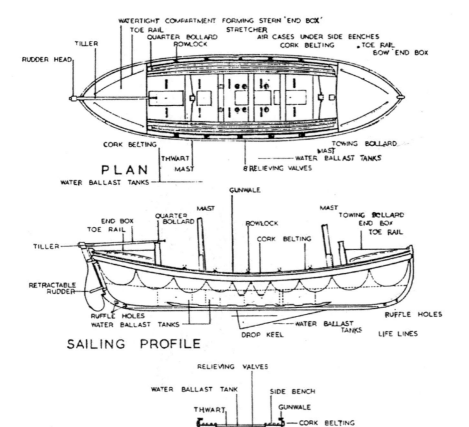

PLAN

SAILING PROFILE

CROSS SECTION AT MIDSHIPS

- If the boat was a self-righting one she had to retain that quality after the engine was fitted, and power had to be cut off in the event of capsize.
- The sailing and pulling qualities of the boat would have to be unaffected and she would have to be unsinkable.
- The engine would have to be simple enough to be controlled by an unskilled member of the crew in an emergency situation.
- The engine must always be ready to start. Winter or summer, even after being idle for some time.

Despite these seemingly impossible requirements, tests began early in 1904 when a nine horse-power engine was fitted to the 38 foot self-righting lifeboat *J. McConnell Hussy*. A speed of six knots was attained with the engine running at 450 rpm and using one and a half gallons of petrol per hour. Taylor engines proved very satisfactory. Sixty or forty horsepower engines were fitted to the larger boats and thirty-five horsepower engines were deemed sufficient for the smaller and self-righting boats. When Taylor engines ceased production the Weyburn engine was accepted as a suitable alternative.

The production of a lifeboat with a cabin was the next major development. Heretofore the only shelter available to the crew or survivors was a sail draped over a spar. Between 1923 and 1925 ten boats with cabins, built to Watson's design, each 45 feet in length, were built. One of these boats was to be assigned to the re-opened Valentia Station in November 1946. Lifeboat design had come a long way since the *Crosby Leonard* was taken off station fifty-six years earlier.

The cabin had seats to accommodate twenty survivors. The hull was of double diagonal planking, being of Honduras mahogany on English oak. The length was 45 feet, the beam 12 feet 6 inches and the displacement tonnage was 20 tons with a full crew and gear on board. Watertight transverse bulkheads divided the boat into seven compartments and ninety-one airtight boxes rendered her unsinkable.

The engine room was made flameproof by means of copper floor and sides. In the event of fire the engine room could be isolated by closing all hatches. Outside the engine room bulkheads and below deck were two petrol tanks which had sufficient capacity for the boat to travel 50 miles at a speed of eight to nine knots.

A canopy protecting the cockpit where the engine controls were situated also provided some protection for the coxswain and crew. Sixteen hand pumps were fitted on deck, enabling pumping out of all compartments in the event of flooding. This design was equipped with a foremast and two sails. All ten boats were fitted with eighty horsepower Weyburn single engines, and in 1929 one of the boats, *John R. Webb*, was re-engined with a diesel engine and became the first diesel-powered lifeboat.

In 1923, the first twin-engined lifeboat, designed by Mr J.R. Barnett, went on station in New Brighton. By 1936 the smallest lifeboat in the fleet was twin engined. Pulling and sailing lifeboats were phased out. The last sailing lifeboat in the fleet was the *William Cantrell Ashley* which remained at New Quay, Cardiganshire until 1948. Along with her replacement – the motor lifeboat RNLB *St Albans* – these were the first lifeboats to be televised in December 1948. *St Albans* was broken up at Arklow in 2005. The last pulling lifeboat *Robert and Ellen Robson* did harbour duty at Whitby until 1957, where she is retained in a museum and in recent years has been launched for fundraising purposes. While this development took place, Valentia was without a lifeboat, but was not without gallant rescues. The *Kerry Sentinel* recalled such a rescue in recounting the events of 14 September 1908:

> A Seine boat and follower from the fishing village of Portmagee shot their seine net inside Valentia Lighthouse about nine o'clock on Monday night. The seine was a large one. By the time the seine was cleared, both boats fully laden with fish had drifted about half a mile outside the harbour. The Seine boat finding it could make no headway against the ebb tide, called on the follower to give them a tow.
>
> This was done and all went well until the harbour entrance was reached, when the boats pulling close to the Beginish shore to avoid the rapid current, got the backwash from the adjacent rocks. The Seine boat, having little free-board was 'swamped'.

The paper told how the crew of the follower hauled on the tow rope until the seine boat crew could board the follower. Another huge backwash swamped the follower, throwing all nineteen men of both crews into the water. Both boats turned turtle and several men clung to them and to the oars. Six men went down. J. Hartnett, captain of the follower said, 'We were more than half an hour in the water, and we saw two boats pulling towards us, they shouted, "Hold on, you are alright".' The following members of our crew were drowned: Pat Kelly, John Devane Senior, John Devane Junior, John O'Sullivan, John Casey and John O'Shea. Poor O'Shea dropped off the oar which he shared with a comrade when the rescuers were at arms length'. The same *Kerry Sentinel* dated 9 December 1908 carried the following report:

> Valentia Disaster Gallantry Awards
> The King has been pleased on the recommendation of the Board of Trade to award Bronze Medals for gallantry in saving life at sea to Michael Cahill, Timothy Cahill, John Cahill, Pat Donoghue, Philip Connell, Timothy Connell, John Sugrue, Con Shea, John Connell, Dan Connell, Michael Falvey, John Connell, Michael Keating, Patrick Sugrue, Patrick Connell, Thomas Lee, John Connell and Peter Donoghue of Knightstown, Valentia, in recognition of their services in rescuing survivors of the fishing boats 'Aughlass' and 'Skelligs' off Tralee on 4th September last. The Board of Trade have awarded the sum of £1.1.0 to each of the fishermen named in recognition of their services on the occasion.

The text of the letter which accompanied the medal to each recipient was as follows:

> Board of Trade,
> Whitehall Gardens,
> December 1908.

Sirs,

I have great pleasure in transmitting to you the accompanying Bronze Medal for gallantry in saving life at sea which His Majesty the King has been pleased, upon my recommendations, to award to you as a mark of appreciation of your services in assisting to rescue the survivors of the crews of the fishing boats 'Aughlass' and 'Skelligs' of Tralee which were swamped while fishing off Valentia, County Kerry on the 14th September last. It affords me much gratification to be the medium of forwarding the medals to you.

I am Sir,

Your obedient servant,

Winston S. Churchill.

What neither the king, the papers, the Board of Trade nor the fishermen could explain was the white boat which spurred the rescuers to the scene by challenging them to a race to the lighthouse as they returned at a leisurely pace. 'The Cahills Seine', as the episode is recalled locally, is now firmly embedded in local folklore.

A memorial plaque was erected in September 2008 to remember this heroic event.

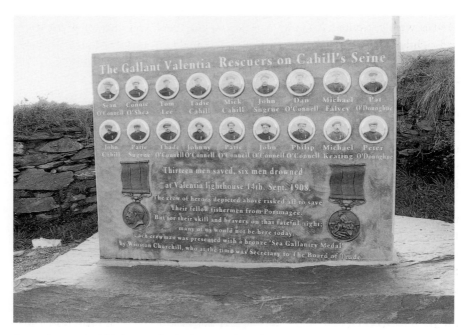

Store pier memorial, Valentia Island. Photo: Dick Robinson.

FOUR

VALENTIA COASTGUARD RADIO & HISTORICAL RESCUES

It was ironic that a few short years later, there was erected, virtually overlooking the scene of the Cahill's Seine disaster, what has become the ears of the eastern Atlantic – Valentia Radio Station. In 1933, the small Norwegian Steamer *Sisto* was in serious trouble far out in the Atlantic Ocean. The tanker *Mobil Oil* and two liners *Aurania* and *New York* were diverted to the scene. While *Aurania* provided a lee and *Mobil Oil* pumped oil to stop the seas breaking and calm them, *New York* effected a rescue. Headlines stated, 'Heroism at Sea', 'Gallant Atlantic Rescue'. Medals were presented, hands shaken, champagne drunk and cigars smoked — and rightly so. That one alert operator in his draughty cliff-top station in Valentia had picked up a very weak SOS and blasted it on powerful transmitters to the rescue ships was totally overlooked.

The operators still work in a building perched on a Valentia Cliff top, albeit in much more comfortable surroundings. They still remain the, 'Cinderellas at the sharp end', for on their vigilance depends the question of effective and timely rescue, or no rescue at all. If the operators may still be occasionally overlooked when the credits for successful rescue are given out, they are never found wanting in their service.

The station opened in Valentia in 1914 under the control of the Admiralty and run by naval personnel. In 1922, the station passed to civilian control under the Inspector of Wireless Telegraphy of the British Post Office and naval personnel were replaced by a civilian staff. In 1950, the stations at Valentia and Malin Head passed to the control of the Irish Government on foot of an agreement between the Irish and British authorities.

Patrick Foran was the first civilian officer-in-charge until his sudden death on 26 July 1952. He was succeeded by Harold Robinson who retired in 1968 and Brendan Sugrue then took over, the first native Valentia islander to do so. In 1993, following Brendan's retirement, Eugene Sullivan was appointed officer-in-charge. Following his retirement in 2004, John Falvey was appointed in an acting capacity and confirmed in the position in 2008. An announcement that

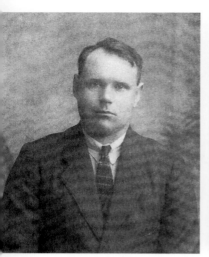 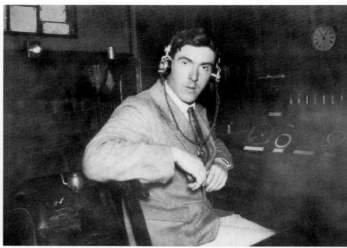

Left: Patrick Foran, 1922. Photo: courtesy of Richard Foran. *Right:* H.H. (Joe) Robinson at Valentia Radio, 1926. Photo: Dick Robinson Collection.

Valentia and Malin Head Radio stations were to be closed was fiercely resisted. A massive media and political campaign bore fruit and in December 2008 the Transport Minister announced that both stations, as well as the one in Dublin would be retained and upgraded.

Valentia Coastguard Radio Staff Past and Present

Bardon, Ian, RIP
Buckley, Tom
Burke, Padd,y RIP
Byrne, Tom
Cahill, Edward, RIP
Campbell, Gerry
Cantillon, Michael, RIP
Carmody, Sean, RIP
Cooper, Francis
Cullen, Frank
Curran, Con (service attendant), RIP
Curtin, Maurice★
Devane, Kevin
Drake, P.
Draper, John★
Egan, Michael
Evans, Robin★

Fahy, Matt
Falvey, John O/C ★
Farren, Michael★
Fitzimons, Patrick, RIP
Foran, Patrick. O/C, RIP
Foy, J.V.
Frawley, Michael, RIP
Geoghegan, Declan
Geoghegan, John★
Grainne, Houlihan (service attendant)
Guiney, Con, RIP
Guirey, Jim★
Healy, Danny (service attendant)★
Heaslip, Ted★
Hogan, Mike
Jennings, Aidan
Kelly, Niall
Kiely, Denis, RIP
Leahy, Joe
Lynch, Francie★
Lynch, Danny★
Lyne, Timothy★
Moroney, P.
O'Brien, Jerry
O'Brien, John★
O'Conno, Willie
O'Connor Michael (service attendant)
O'Keefe, Bill, RIP
O'Sullivan, Danny (engine attendant), RIP
O'Neill, John H.(Johno), RIP
O'Shea, Michael David, RIP
O'Sullivan, Brendan, RIP
O'Sullivan, John★
O'Sullivan, Tom
Orpen, Russell★
Quigley, John (services attendant)
Robinson, Harold (Joe) O/C
Shrouder, Stevie
Sugrue, Brendan O/C
Sullivan, Eugene O/C

(★) Current Staff.

Wireless telegraphy has since been augmented by radio telephony. VHF was introduced on 1 June 1983 with repeater stations along the coast in 1987 extending the range and eliminating many black spots where reception was impossible. In 1951, came a rather bizarre reversal of roles whereby the lifeboat was enabled to render a service to Valentia Radio Station! St Stephen's Day 1951 was to see the beginning of a storm which whipped the Atlantic to a fury which would not subside for several weeks. On the night of 19 December the seas were mountainous and wave after giant wave crashed on the roof of the cliff top radio station. Eventually the roof gave way and water swamped in, wrecking the equipment. For the first time in its history the ears of the Atlantic had been deafened. As a contingency plan, the equipment at the Cork Radio School had to be geared up to give limited emergency cover while the station at Valentia was repaired but such were the conditions that no ferryboat could put to sea and the lifeboat had to launch to take three radio operators to Cahirciveen so that they could make the trip to Cork with all haste. The entry on the station service board '30.12.1951, Valentia Radio, Gave Help', always prompts the question among the uninitiated, 'How does a lifeboat assist a Radio Station?' Would that more people would be aware of how much the Radio Station assists the lifeboat!

From 1972, the Marine Rescue Co-Ordination Centre had been a function of the Air Traffic Services and was located at Shannon. It was run on an agency basis for the Department of the Marine, with Michael Cotter being the officer-in-charge. Its purpose was the co-ordination of available rescue units to maximize effectiveness to ensure safe and speedy assistance to mariners and ships.

The particular responsibilities of MRCC were:
- Seeking all relevant information from appropriate sources regarding any incident.
- Assessing what facilities are needed to deal with the incident.
- Ascertaining from a vessel involved in the operation, its location, conditions and intentions.
- Designating where appropriate and advising an On-Scene Commander or Coordinator Surface Search.
- Requesting special action of any vessel involved in the operation.
- Requesting assistance of aircraft if appropriate through the relevant Rescue Coordination Centre.
- Deciding in consultation with other authorities, when lifesaving action is complete or when to terminate an unsuccessful search.

Rescue Units at the disposal of MRCC at Shannon are:
- RNLI Lifeboats.
- Coast Lifesaving Stations.
- Irish Air Corps helicopters and search aircraft.

- MRCC will also avail of the assistance of Irish Naval Service Vessels.
- Shipping in search/distress area.
- Civil Aircraft overlying the relevant area.
- Coastal Garda Stations.
- Irish Lights officers or lighthouses.
- Harbour and Pilotage authorities.
- Qualified officers manning MRCC on a 24 hour basis.

In 1993, the Marine Rescue Coordination Centre's role was handed over to the Irish Marine Emergency Service. They had three bases, at Valentia, Malin Head and Dublin. Each station had a dual role as Coastal Radio and Search and Rescue Coordination Centre. A fax from MRCC Shannon to all agencies ended with the words 'Last out switch off the lights'.

In 2000, the service became known as the Irish Coastguard Service. The purpose of the Coastguard Service is:

> To reduce the loss of life within the Irish Search and Rescue Region and on rivers, lakes and waterways and to protect the quality of the marine environment within the Irish Pollution Responsibility Zone, harbours and Maritime Local Authority areas and to preserve property. To promote safety standards, and by doing so, prevent, as far as possible, the loss of life at sea and on inland waters and other areas, and to provide an effective emergency response service.

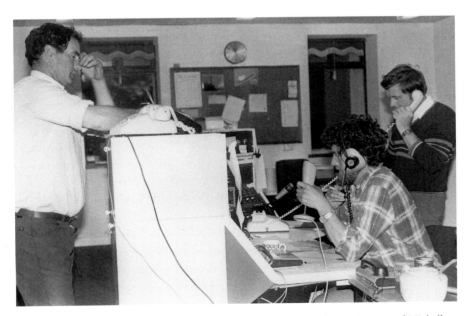

Valentia Radio staff in action during the Air India crash of 1985. Photo: courtesy of Michelle Cooper Galvin.

The Irish Coastguard (IRCG) makes up one arm of the Maritime Safety Services, the other being the Maritime Safety Directorate. Both arms are due to merge into a new 'one stop shop' Agency for all maritime safety matters.

Before the native Government took over, the coast was covered by the British Coastguard. This service was withdrawn when the take over occurred. Whatever the reasons, the situation whereby a trained and attentive human eye monitored the entire coast had disappeared. All the current technical navigational and electronic aids are magnificent, but the observant human eye is also a necessary ingredient.

At Valentia, the Coastguard had two stations and dwellings. One was at the western end of the island, facing Portmagee, near the bridge, where the houses still stand. The other was at Knightstown, where Peter Street and the Coastal Terrace were Coastguard residences. The operational enclosure at Knightstown still stands and retains the name 'The Watch House'. Coastguards stationed at Valentia were decorated by the RNLI on two occasions, being awarded a total of six silver medals. The details have been gleaned from contemporary newspapers as RNLI records are not available. On Saturday 6 December 1828 a tremendous hurricane struck the west coast of Ireland. One Limerick ship, inward bound from London, was stranded at Moneypoint near Kilrush, with the loss of keel and forefoot and had to discharge her cargo there. At Limerick, a port 50 miles inland from the Atlantic fury, the *Irene* of London lost two boats at Beagh Castle. The *Quebec Packet* lost an anchor and several fathoms of cable. The *Industrious, Master Davis*, had her bow stove in at Russells Quay and the *Clio* of Alloa lost her jib boom. The *Veronica* of Belfast, Eustace her master, was on passage from Belfast to Charlestown in the United States. A 350 ton brig, she carried a cargo of salt and coal. She was driven up Dingle Bay throughout Saturday night and ran ashore at Inch Bar on Sunday morning. She was the property of Messrs Halloran of Belfast and had sailed from that city on 10 November 1828:

> The entire crew and passengers were saved with the exception of a woman named Jennings who was swept overboard. Their safety is altogether owing (under Providence) to the Waterguards of Minard, under Mr. Roe – to Francis Roe Esq. of Minard, most laudably assisted by several of his tenancy – and to Captain Bowie of Dingle, Commander of the Coastguard', the paper concluded.

While the details of their part in this rescue are not specifically detailed in the papers of the time, five Coastguards attached to Valentia Station, William Rowe, J. Renowden, William Marx, Richard Jeffers and Richard Hanning, were each voted a silver medal for gallantry by the Committee of Management of RNLI on the 24 December 1828.

On 19 November 1850, the drama at sea was west of Kilshannig. The 263-ton brig *Enrichetta* of Naples was inward bound from Barletta in southern Italy to Limerick. She was driven ashore in horrendous weather. John Town Chief Officer of Coastguard, with other men to help him, waded into the surf and took off ten of the twelve-man crew. He was awarded the silver medal by the RNLI. Like Mr Kearney White, Mr Town already held two silver medals for gallantry.

On 12 March 1847 the brig *Henry and Sarah* was wrecked west of Dover. Mr Town launched the Coastguard galley and with a crew of four rescued the master of the ship and seven men. On 21/22 December 1849 in a raging storm the Danish galliot *Margaretta Sabreana* was wrecked off Romney Hay, Folkestone. After launching the coastguard galley and rowing to windward of the casualty they were driven back. They launched again at daybreak and took two men off the masthead. After returning to shore to bail out their vessel he put out again and saved a further two men.

Inch Strand was again the scene for the rescue from the *Florence Graham* of six people in January 1861. The *Florence Graham*, an 870-ton brig, was inward bound from Brara River, Vento in West Africa to her home port of Liverpool. Owned by Messrs Halloran and Cookson of Mersey Street in that city, she carried a cargo of palm oil. In extremely poor conditions, the *Florence Graham* had her pumps manned day and night for ten days before the storm caught her. It drove her from a course which should have taken her up the Irish Sea. Instead she was driven into Dingle Bay and flung ruthlessly on Inch Bar. The captain and six men took to a boat which capsized twenty yards from the wreck. Although the captain and another man gained footing, all were lost, swept away by receding waves.

The mate tried to swim ashore with a rope and a lifebuoy but had to be hauled back onto the wreck where he died from exhaustion, cold and exposure within a matter of minutes. The wreck broke in two. One end of it was driven up the beach with seven men clinging to it, of whom five were swept away and lost. One of the other two was saved by Thomas Kennedy of Annascaul. Coastguard Hugh Cooper of Valentia Coastguard Station, chief boatman and his crew, including Coastguard Twomey of Minard, launched their boat into the violent seas and snatched the other man from the wreck. The remaining survivors, three men, were saved by sub-constables McCarthy and Rice of Annascaul, who, with Timothy Moriarty, waded into the surf up to their armpits. The survivors were so exhausted that they had to be carried on people's backs to the house of the local doctor, Kane, where they were treated. In all, twelve people had lost their lives. The vessel became a total loss. Three crew with scurvy were confined to their quarters where they died. Most of the ship's cargo was saved. The fact that no effort was made to plunder or loot the wreck was commented on favourably in the *Kerry Evening Post* of Saturday 26 January 1861. Bastable Hilliard of Dingle, Lloyds Agent, took charge of the wreck. On 4 April 1861 the Committee of Management of the RNLI voted the silver medal for gallantry to Coastguard Hugh Cooper of Valentia.

There were many changes since the closure of the Valentia Lifeboat Station. Perhaps the most significant was on the political landscape. Ireland was divided

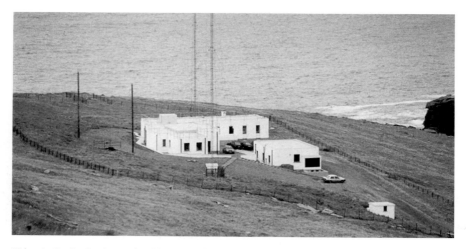

Valentia Radio Station today. Photo: Dick Robinson.

by the treaty of 6 December 1921 which was ratified by the Irish Government on 7 January 1922. Twenty-six Counties became 'The Irish Free State' while six remained within the United Kingdom. After correspondence between the Provisional Government of the Irish Free State and the Royal National Lifeboat Institution a meeting was arranged. A deputation from the Committee of Management of the RNLI met with the Minister for Home Affairs in Dublin in October 1922. Following a request by the Provisional Government, it was agreed that the RNLI would continue to provide the lifeboat service in the Free State.

The RNLI today still operates in the Republic as a charity. Perhaps the most highly visible support for some twenty years was the relief lifeboat RNLB *Hibernia* (ON 1150 52.44). She entered the relief fleet in September 1989 and was withdrawn in February 2007. She had launched on service 315 times and saved forty-four lives. By passing 'The Irish Sailors and Soldiers Land Trust Act 1988' the Irish Government, who were the trustees of that fund, transferred the funds to purchase the relief lifeboat to the RNLI.

The repeal of the External Relations Act of 1948, the creation of the Irish Republic in 1949 or the Good Friday Agreement of 1988 had no effect on the manner in which the RNLI operates.

During the Second World War the RNLI made provisions for rescue of airmen whose planes crashed into the sea off the Irish Coast. As virtually no lifeboats were built during the war, open motor boats were employed as 'Auxiliary Life Boats'. They operated from thirteen ports in the following locations: Ballinskelligs, Co. Kerry; Blacksod, Co. Mayo; Castletownbere, Co. Cork; Courtown, Co. Wexford; Dingle, Co. Kerry; Downings, Co. Donegal; Gola Island, Co. Donegal: Inishbofin, Co. Galway; Malin Head, Co. Donegal; Teelin, Co. Donegal; Meenlaragh, Co. Donegal; Tory Island, Co. Donegal; Valentia, Co. Kerry.

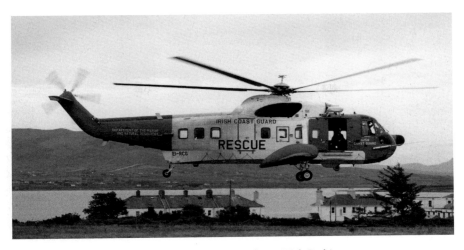

Coastguard helicopter touching down at Valentia. Photo: Dick Robinson.

A lifeboat was made available at Killybegs. The St Peter Port Lifeboat had been in Cowes, Isle of Wight, for overhaul. The Channel Islands were invaded by the Germans so their lifeboat *Queen Victoria* could not return to station. She was assigned to Killybegs. She remained there from 1941 to 1945, when the station was closed. She was credited with saving four lives at Killybegs. She returned to St Peter Port in 1945 and served there and in the relief fleet until 1958. After service she became a yacht and was destroyed by fire.

List of Services by the Auxiliary Lifeboat *St Bernard* at Valentia between 1943 and 1946

(Courtesy of The Lifeboat Digital Achive and Liz Cook, Editor of *The Lifeboat* journal.) The *St Bernard* was the last of the Auxiliary lifeboats to remain in service and remained so until November 1946 when Valentia Lifeboat Station reopened:

At about midnight on 16/17 April 1943 the *St Bernard* was at sea fishing. The crew saw distress signals form a fishing vessel four miles north of the Skelligs Rock. She found the *Tigileen* of Portmagee with a crew of four on board. Her engine had broken drown. There was a heavy sea running. The *St Bernard* took the casualty in tow. The tow rope parted several times and finally was trebled and held. When about two miles north of Bray Head the *Tigileen* started her engine and was able to proceed under her own power.

On 9 December the fishing boat *Naomh Sean* was reported to be disabled 5 miles north-west of Valentia Radio Point. There was a strong south-easterly wind and a rough sea. The *St Bernard* came to her assistance, put a line on board and towed her to Valentia harbour.

On 27 February 1944 an aeroplane was reported in the sea at the Skelligs. The *St Bernard* put to sea at 4 a.m. There was a strong north-easterly wind and a heavy sea. It was bitterly cold. Conditions were so severe that the pump had to be kept going all the time on the boat. After an extensive search, with nothing being found, the *St Bernard* returned to base. She had a difficult time in entering Portmagee which she reached at 7.15 p.m.

Patty Lynch, The Lotts, Valentia was in the local hospital in 1993. He was mentioned in *The Kerryman* in that year as 'the last surviving member of the crew of the auxillary lifeboat'. He recalled the terrible conditions they had endured in the above service.

On 19 August 1990 Valentia lifeboat led a flotilla of local craft out of the harbour and wreaths were laid in the sea in memory of the American airmen.

On 1 April 1944 the Coast Lifesaving Service reported a vessel in distress at Bray Head. The *St Bernard* set out at 8 a.m. At the same time a cable ship took the casualty in tow. The cable ship handed the tow of the 'Rearcha Na Fairrige' over to the *St Bernard* within the harbour and she was towed to the pier.

On 25 October 1944 the *St Bernard* was returning from fishing. She sighted flares 3 miles north-west-west of the Wireless Point. She found the fishing boat *Naomh Sean* of Caherciveen with a crew of four broken down. She took the casualty in tow to Renard pier.

On 7 November 1944 while returning from fishing the *St Bernard* saw a flare 2 miles north-east of Bray Head. There was a strong ebb tide and a heavy sea. She found the fishing vessel *Spray* of Valentia with six people on board with a fouled propeller. A Caherciveen fishing boat had attempted a tow but had to abandon it because of heavy seas. The *St Bernard* secured a towline and towed her to safety at Valentia.

On 22 May 1946 the *St Bernard* was returning from the fishing grounds as the conditions were too bad for fishing. At about 9 p.m. she found the fishing boat *Dun Ciara* of Portmagee with a crew of four broken down 3 miles north-west of Bray Head. There was a strong south-south-east wind and a rough sea. She took the casualty in tow, the tow parted five times in the conditions. The casualty was finally landed at Portmagee pier at 1 a.m.

FIVE

VALENTIA LIFEBOAT STATION RE-OPENED

On 20 November 1946 Valentia Lifeboat Branch was formally reconstituted and the station reopened. Commander Dutton, the District Inspector of Lifeboats in Ireland, chaired a meeting at the Royal Hotel at 6.30 p.m. on that date. Present were Mr Scott RNLI District Engineer, Mr Webb District Surveyor, Very Revd James Kennedy, Parish Priest, W. Shanahan, T. O'Driscoll, P. Foran (O/C Valentia Radio), F. A. Whittlesey, H. O'Sullivan, K. O'Driscoll, J. Shanahan and T. R. Stewart, the honorary secretary.

Boats Officers were appointed as follows: coxswain – Jeremiah O'Connell, second coxswain – James (Dev) Lynch, mechanic – James Flanagan, assistant mechanic – John Dore. Flanagan was in fact an RNLI fleet mechanic and in accordance with usual practice would remain at the station until John Dore had

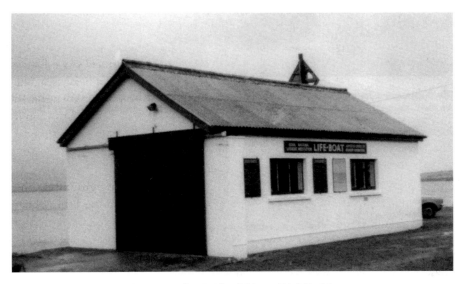

The lifeboat store at Knightstown, Valentia Island. Photo: Dick Robinson.

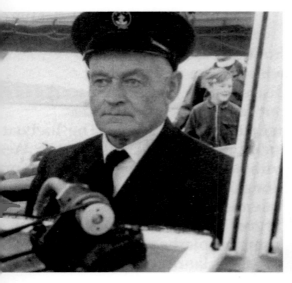

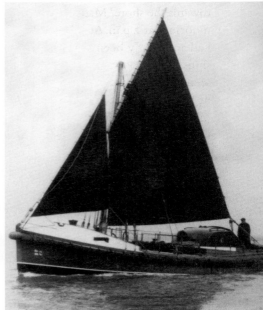

Above: Coxswain Jeremiah O'Connell. Photo: courtesy of Valentia Heritage Centre.

Right: RNLB. *C&S*. Photo: courtesy of the RNLI.

sufficiently trained to take over as mechanic. It was somewhat inappropriate in this case as Dore had served his time in the Kelvin Engineering Works in Scotland and knew as much as any living being about marine engines, or any engines.

RNLB *C&S* was the first lifeboat assigned to the station. She was a 45 foot Watson class lifeboat powered by a single eighty horse-power Weyburn engine. She was funded from a gift of Mr Coats and a legacy of Miss Smart. Her Official Number was 690. She was built at the yard of S.E. Saunders in Cowes, Isle of Wight in 1925 at a cost of £8,424. She served at Dunmore East; Pwllheli and in the reserve fleet before coming to Valentia.

On her delivery journey to Valentia the lifeboat was under the command of Irish District Inspector, Lieutenant Commander W.L.G. Dutton, calling to Ballycotton on 15 November 1946 for fuel and rest. She launched on service twice and saved no lives. She was last reported as a yacht *Caradoc* at Victoria B.C. Canada in July 1985. The first service call at the Valentia Station was on 26 December 1946.

False alarm with Good Intent

'Dingle Coast Lifesaving Depot report that a Spanish Trawler has been sighted flying a distress signal 3 miles north-west of Keownglass Point and is drifting fast towards the shore.' Maroons were fired at 1.47 p.m. and the lifeboat *C&S* slipped moorings at 2 p.m. At 5 p.m. the lifeboat located a Starboard Hand buoy, which had apparently been at sea for some time. As the search had revealed no other ships in distress this was accepted to be what the Coast Lifesaving Depot had seen. On returning to harbour the seas were such that the moorings could not be picked up. The lifeboat was refuelled and left at the Quay Wall. Crew on the first service launch were: Flanagan J., Dore J., Walsh D., Murphy J., Murphy P., O'Leary, Sugrue P, McCrohen P., Stewart T., (Cox).

Lifeboat as a Hearse

On 12 January 1947, a request was received from the Superintendent of the Garda Siochána at Dingle for the removal of a body from the Blasket Islands for a post-mortem. No other suitable boat was available in the weather prevailing at the time, the lifeboat *C&S* slipped moorings at 12.40 a.m. and proceeded to Dingle to embark the local Sergeant. They proceeded to the Blaskets, embarked the body and landed it at Dingle. The lifeboat was back at station at 1.55 am on the 13 January. So widespread were the storms of those January days the lifeboat at Aith in the Shetland Islands spent the 12 January bringing food to Papa Stour Island, cut off for three weeks.

In 1947, the lifeboat *BASP* was assigned to Valentia and served from 1947 to 1951. Built in 1924 by J.S. White of Cowes under ON 687 she was an identical

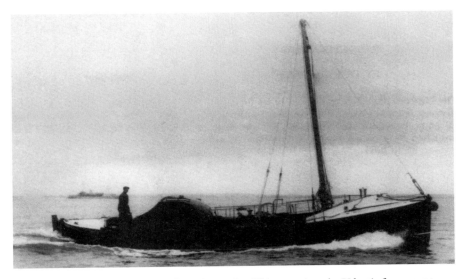

RNLB *BASP*, a second forty-five-foot Watson class lifeboat stationed at Valentia from 1947 to 1951. This boat will be a permanent exhibit at the Chatham Dockyard Display. Photo: courtesy of the RNLI.

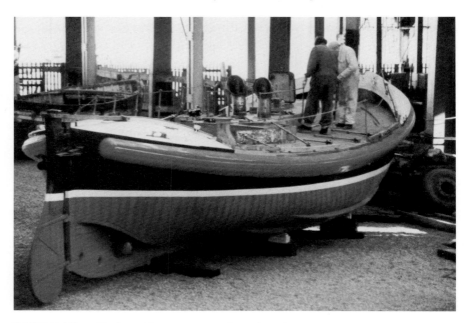

RNLB *BASP* at Chatham. Photo: courtesy of Peter Woolhouse.

sister ship of *C&S*. She was funded from legacies of Mrs Smart; Mrs Price, Mr Blackburn and Mrs Armstrong and cost £7,519. She had served at Yarmouth, Isle of Wight, Falmouth and in the reserve fleet before coming to Valentia. The *BASP* is now in the Historical Lifeboat Collection at Chatham in London. She is currently being restored and is part of the permanent display entitled 'Lifeboat' at the Historic Dockyard.

Flares Investigated

On 18 September 1947 at 6.30 a.m. the honorary secretary was called by the No. 1 man of the Coast Lifesaving Service and informed that the following message had been received from the Local Garda Barracks; 'A message has been received from Caherciveen Garda Barracks that distress flares had been seen to the west of the Skelligs Islands'.

The *BASP* slipped moorings at 7 a.m. At 7.04 a.m. contact was made with Valentia Wireless Station and the following information was received. At 2.35 a.m. Skelligs Wireless had reported White Flares seen at 51.35 north. and 10.40 west approximately 13 miles south of the Skelligs. A course was set accordingly. At 8.57 a.m. contact was made with the Skelligs Light House. They had not reported anything to Valentia Wireless Station. At 9.45 a.m. Valentia Wireless Station relayed that a mistake had been made. The position given had been that of a ship reporting the presence of white distress flares north of the Skelligs. The course was immediately altered and a sweep was from approximately 18 miles south–west to 9 miles north of the Skelligs. In the search area a motor ship, two British trawlers and a private yacht under full canvas were sighted. All would have been within sight of the area where the flares were reported and they themselves were not in distress. The lifeboat returned to base. Four tins of soup and one tin of chocolate were expended, 'although the hours at sea were short it will be appreciated that these men were out before breakfast' remarked the honorary secretary.

The honorary secretary wrote the following:

Service 18 September 1947

I would like to bring to your notice the following observations with regard to the system adopted for the call out of the lifeboat on this occasion. I have tried to piece together what actually took place from the time the Original Message was sent from the British Ship 'Salacia'. It would appear that this ship sighted flares sometime around 02.00 hours and that she informed 'Val. Wireless. Val. Wireless informed the Department of Industry and Commerce in Dublin. Who in turn contacted Cork, who in turn telephoned Caherciveen and tried to get in touch with Lloyds agent there (who, by the way retired last December and no one new has been appointed). The Caherciveen Garda were then informed and they telephoned Valentia Garda who called out the No. 1 Man of the Coast Lifesaving Service who at last called me.

I have obtained (Unofficially) from the Garda Barracks here a copy of the message which they received, eventually. 4.11 a.m. (GMT) Valentia Radio Priority at 03.06 (GMT) Addressed Valentia Radio.

Message begins:

'Several White Rockets seen North True from the Great Skelligs Light. Our position at 02.35 hrs 51.35N 10.40W. Master. British Ship, 'Salacia'."

It appears to me that a great amount of 'red tape' is holding up these messages.

Valentia Wireless are connected by a 24 hour telephone to Mr. Foran's house (Manager of Station) which is in the village here, also the Garda are on a 24 hour telephone together with the No. 1 Man Coast Live Saving and our own Coxswain. I might mention here that no telephone was ever installed in my residence. This means that before I can receive a message it has to go through several persons and as the message passes from one to another not only is time being lost but mistakes, additions or important information is being left out of the original message. I would suggest that if at all possible, both the Wireless Station and the Garda be informed that should the lifeboat be required the Hon. Sec. should be told first or at the earliest possible opportunity.

T/R. Stewart.

Hon. Sec.

Overdue Fishing Boats

In June 1948, the reserve lifeboat *City of Bradford 1* (ON 680) was on temporary duty at Valentia. The fact that she had no wireless on the 17 June 1948 led to a report that makes interesting reading as reported by Mr T.R. Stewart, the honorary secretary. A Practice having been arranged for the morning of the 17 June (1948) reserve lifeboat ON 680 left her moorings under Coxswain O'Connell and a full crew at 10 a.m.

At 10.20 a.m. a telephone call was received by the honorary secretary from the Post Office at Portmagee stating that one of the fishing boats which had put to sea the previous evening had not returned and anxiety was felt for their wellbeing. Full details were received as to the position that this boat was last seen, i.e. 3 a.m. 2 miles north-west of Great Skellig Island.

The course which ON 680 was to have taken was through the southern entrance so Portmagee was instructed to have a boat stand by and as soon as the lifeboat was sighted to stop her and inform her of the casualty.

The honorary secretary immediately went to Bray Head Look Out Post to see if there was any sign of the missing boat, so that he could semaphore directions to the Coxswain. There being no sign, he returned to the Watch House (Lifeboat Station) and contacted the following by telephone; Ballinskelligs Post Office, Derrynane, Waterville, Dursey Island and made arrangements with the Shore Dwellings of the Irish Lights to keep an hourly watch by telephone (radio) with the Skelligs Lighthouse. He then got in touch with Father O'Donovan (Baltimore Lifeboat Station) to stand by should they fail to locate this boat before she had drifted too far south.

Another run as made by the honorary secretary to Bray Head and the lifeboat could be seen heading south for the Bull Rock, but as he failed to see the missing fishing boat in the vicinity he returned and asked Valentia Radio to broadcast a message to all shipping in this area to keep a look out for a 28 foot fishing boat painted blue with a yellow top band, containing a crew of four men, believed to have been 2 miles north-west of the Skelligs at 3 a.m. This was put on air immediately. A telephone call was put through to Captain Frayne in Dublin to see if it could be arranged to have an Army Scout Plane search the locality.

A short time afterwards the Deparment of Defence were on the telephone to say that a plane would put out from Rynanna and would circle this station three times and then head off in the direction of the casualty. As several other boats had left in the morning to help in the search I requested each port to try and recall any boats that were in their vicinity, also asked the Skelligs to hoist their flag in the hope that the lifeboat would see it and give them a message to return to base for re-fuelling and to wait for the aeroplane.

The lifeboat during this period made a wide search from the Skelligs to north of the Bull. From there she made for Hog Island and back out towards the Skelligs

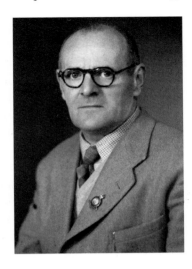

Kieran O'Driscoll, Hon. Secretary of Valentia Lifeboat 1949 to 1967. Photo: courtesy of Mary Sheedy (*née* O'Driscoll).

when she spotted the flag and received the message to return, heading in from the Skelligs she spotted three small boats close under Bolus Cliffs and identified one as the missing boat and the other two as boats which had put to sea earlier in the morning she escorted them in through the southern entrance and when they were safe in Portmagee she returned to her base.

All concerned were immediately notified that the missing boat was now safe. The aeroplane was stopped just as she was about to take off. Great concern was felt from the beginning as both the owners and crew of this boat are considered first-class fishermen and that unless something drastic had happened they would have returned before 7 a.m.

The cable ship *Marie Louise Mackay*, which was working in Ballinskelligs Bay, wirelessed to Valentia Radio Station offering assistance, but by this time the missing boat had been located and was on her way back to port.

Mr P. Casey was interviewed and it was ascertained that he was fishing off the Skelligs, having hauled his nets was returning when he developed engine trouble about one mile west of Bray Head. The small sail which he carried was of no use to beat to windward and as the tides were so strong he was unable to make any headway so spent the night at the oars keeping her off the land and eventually was picked up about 4 miles west of Scarriff Island by one of the Portmagee fishing boats.

On 5 January 1949, Mr Stewart resigned as honorary secretary Mr Kieran O'Driscoll was appointed in his place Mr J. Shanahan being assistant honory secretary.

A local tragedy

On 21st January 1950 the fishing boat 'San Pedro' was reported overdue. The lifeboat BASP launched at 22.35 hours and searched from an area 3 miles North West of the Lighthouse, where the vessel had last been seen sailing toward Bray

Head. The search continued throughout the 22nd. Fenit lifeboat was asked to search North of the Blaskets. On the 23rd the lifeboat searched with the assistance of an army plane. The three men (two of whom were lifeboat men) were presumed lost and the search was called off.

Skelligs Lighthouse Relieved

In March 1950, the lighthouses at Skelligs and Tearaght were overdue for relief. At the request of the Commissioners of Irish Lights, the *BASP* sailed at 10 a.m. on 24 March for the Skelligs as the keepers had reported that relief was possible. The Tearaght reported that relief should be possible at 3.30 p.m. (low water) the station boarding boat was taken in tow extra crew were taken to man the boarding boat. The Skelligs was relieved at 12.40 p.m. and the lifeboat sailed for the Tearaght. Arriving at 3.35 p.m. rough seas and a force seven south-easterly wind made safe relief too great a risk.

Tearaght Lighthouse Relieved

On 26 March 1950, a message was received from the Tearaght that relief would be possible. Relief keepers and provisions were embarked and the lifeboat BASP with boarding boat and extra crew sailed at 10.10 a.m. and reached the rock at 12.30 a.m. Stores were landed by derrick from the boarding boat. The lifeboat then proceeded to the North Landing and embarked the liberty keepers. The lifeboat was back at Valentia at 4.15 p.m.

The honorary secretary recommended that £2 (the cost of hiring a local boat) be charged to Irish Lights (who in such cases refund the costs of the services) towards maintenance of the boarding boat. Telegrams in respect of 24 March cost 5s 9d and for 26 March cost 3s.

Temporary Lifeboats at the Station

Between 1946 and 1951 inclusive, the *City of Bradford I*, launched five times on service saving eight lives. She became the workboat *Hammer* with Wimpys. Her present whereabouts are unknown. On 12 March 1951 Mr P. Foran (O/C, Valentia Radio) was appointed assistant honorary secretary RNLI in London had requested a change of assistant honorary secretary as Mr Shanahan was away for long periods.

SIX

A TWIN-ENGINED LIFEBOAT – THE *AED*

In February 1951, Valentia received a twin-engine lifeboat, the first at the station. She was RNLB *AED*, 51 foot Barnett class lifeboat which had been built in 1929 at a cost of £10,119 and was previously stationed at Holyhead. There she launched on service eighty-four times and saved 153 lives. She was powered by two Weyburn C.E.6 engines. She would now feature in many Valentia rescues.

Four People Saved

On 5 May 1951, at 9.10 a.m. a telephone message was received by the honorary secretary that the open motor boat *Pride of Caherciveen* was overdue by eight hours returning from the fishing grounds. The *AED* launched at 9.30 a.m. The boat was found at 11.30 a.m 5 miles north-west of Bray Head. Its crew of four (including D. Walsh second coxswain of the lifeboat) had battled a force seven easterly wind for a marathon eight hours. The motorboat had been blown 11 miles out to sea. The totally exhausted crew were brought on board the lifeboat and given soup. Their boat was towed to Valentia.

Blasket Islands Receive Storm Relief

A four-week period of worsening weather conditions had made landing at the Blaskets impossible for boats and army planes. At the request of the County Manager, via the Honorary Secretary Kieran O'Driscoll, the lifeboat was instructed to land supplies for the island's twenty-eight inhabitants at 11.30 a.m. on 4 January 1952.

The *AED* slipped her mooring as 12.15 a.m. and proceeded to Renard pier. Here Mr O'Mahony of the Local Authority was embarked. The lifeboat returned to Knightstown pier. Enough food and medical supplies for three weeks were

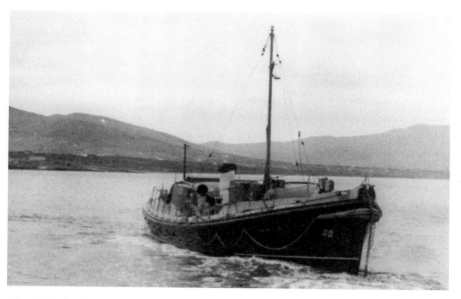

The *AED*, the first twin-engined lifeboat at Valentia from 1951 to 1957. Photo: courtesy of
the *Cork Examiner*.

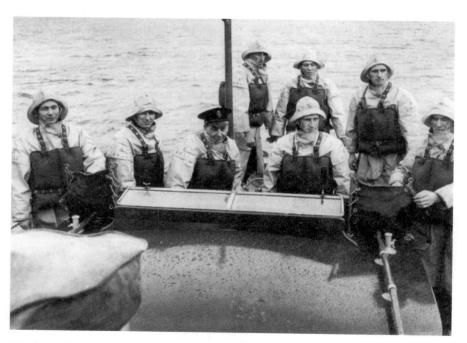

Members of Valentia Lifeboat Crew in early 1950s. Front row, from left to right: Paud Murphy,
Charlie O'Connell, John Dore (mechanic), Dodie Walsh (assistant coxswain) and Padgen
Murphy. Back row: Jack Sugrue, Sean Casey and Diarmuid Walsh. Photo: courtesy of the
RNLI.

embarked. Dr O'Driscoll came on board. There was a north-west gale with hail showers. There was an ebb tide. An extra crewman was taken to assist in manning the boarding boat at the Blaskets. Arriving at the Blaskets at 4 p.m the supplies were landed by 4.50 p.m. in very rough conditions. The lifeboat returned to Valentia at 7.30 p.m. and was refuelled and ready for service at 8 p.m.

Because of a previous error in payment to the institution, the honorary secretary insisted on being given a written guarantee stating that all costs incurred in the provision of the service would be paid by the local authority. This was forwarded to HQ with the return of service.

Mr Foran died suddenly on 26 July 1952. He was succeeded in the position of O/C Valentia Radio and assistant honorary secretary of the lifeboat by H.H. (Joe) Robinson late in 1952.

A Long Search for a French Trawler

On 13 May 1953 Valentia Radio intercepted a distress message from the French trawler *Liberator* of Camaret. She had lost her propeller and she gave her position as 3 miles south of the Blasket Islands and 13 miles north-west by west from the lifeboat station. The *Liberator* was a trawler of 58 tons and carried a crew of nine.

The lifeboats' honorary secretary, Kieran O'Driscoll, received the news at 4.15 p.m. and maroons were fired. At 4.40 p.m. the lifeboat *AED* slipped her moorings with Coxwain Jeremiah O'Connell in command. The sea was rough and confused, there was continuous drizzle and a strong south-south-east wind. Visibility was poor, sometimes nil. The lifeboatmen, wet, cold and hungry, took up positions along the deck so as to maintain a constant visual chain as they ploughed through the seas of the Blaskets archipelago, they received four different positions.

The trawler gave her position, with reference to the Blaskets as, 'west by west by a quarter southwest, anchored in fifty-two fathoms of water in a dense fog'. The position meant nothing to the non-French speaking operators at Valentia Radio, and even when they enlisted the assistance of British Stations at Land's End, Niton and north Foreland, four different possible interpretations of the cryptic position of the casualty emerged. These positions varied from 3 miles south of the Blaskets to 10 miles north-west. After searching all the given positions with still no trace of the trawler. Coxswain O'Connell decided to search all the areas where the crew knew from experience that fifty-two fathoms of water would be found.

At 12.30 a.m. on 14 May 1953 the *Liberator* was found by the lifeboat. She was lying in the trough of a confused sea and rolling heavily. It was pitch dark, with a south-east gale. The trawler had no boat. Having watched the behaviour of the trawler, the coxswain, after consultation with the crew, decided that towing the trawler would be safer all round than to try and go alongside to take off the crew. By sign language the plan was conveyed to and understood by the French captain.

Coxswain O'Connell brought the lifeboat in close under the stern of the violently rolling trawler and, after receiving a line, the heavy manila cable was passed. Having secured the tow, the best course had to be decided. Because of the strong flood tide the coxswain considered going north of the islands. Eventually it was decided that the best course to take was to steer south-eastwards and pass south of the islands, back to Valentia. The best speed that could be made in the prevailing conditions was three knots. The *Liberator* was berthed at Knightstown Quay at 8.05 a.m. The lifeboat was back at moorings refueled and ready for service at 9.45 a.m. Following this service the RNLI awarded their thanks on vellum to Coxswain Jeremiah O'Connell, 'for the sound reasoning and judgment which he exercised and the determination and initiative he showed' on the occasion.

The French Ambassador in Dublin expressed his thanks, stating that 'The generous gesture made by Valentia Branch of the Royal National Lifeboat Institution is greatly appreciated and worthy of its long standing tradition and devotion'. The owners of the trawler made gifts to the RNLI and to the lifeboat crew.

Two English Girls Rescued

On 16 September 1953, while the coxswain, mechanics and honorary secretary were on board the lifeboat at her moorings, Coxswain O'Connell saw his punt, which he had lent to two English girls capsize. The boat was about a mile and a half from the moorings. The lifeboat *AED* proceeded immediately and eighteen minutes later rescued the two girls and recovered the punt.

Milford Haven Trawler and Crew Saved

In very rough seas and snow showers on 28 February 1954 the honorary secretary was informed by Valentia Radio that the trawler *River Spey* of Milford Haven was leaking badly and required urgent assistance. She was 15 miles south-west of the Tearaght Light. The lifeboat *AED* slipped moorings at 6.40 a.m. The seas were rough with a north-east wind force six to eight. On reaching the vessel the lifeboat aided its captain in attempting to save his vessel, by escorting it to Valentia. At the harbour Coxswain O'Connell, also the local pilot, boarded the vessel. She was substantially down by the stern. She was beached off Knightstown pier and her twelve crew were landed at the quay.

Local Trawler Aground

The great shelter of Valentia harbour had appeared on mariners' books as far back as the fifteenth century. But even here the Atlantic storms can penetrate with vengeance and venom. On 26 November 1954, lifeboat Secretary Kieran O'Driscoll received a phone call to say that the *Ros Airgead* registered in Dublin but owned and skippered by Christy O'Shea of Valentia was aground on the White Horse Rocks, south of the Caherciveen River and needed help urgently. Maroons were fired at 7.20 p.m. and by 7.30 p.m. a full crew had mustered at the lifeboat store. A full gale was blowing from the north-west. The tide at half ebb was at its strongest and the sea was extremely rough.

The crew set out in the rowing boat from the beach with two men to each oar. Three times they were thrown back onto the beach. On the fourth attempt and two hours after assembling they boarded the lifeboat at 9.30 p.m. The lifeboat *AED* reached the White Horse Rocks at 10 p.m. and began to search. At 10.27 p.m. Valentia Radio reported that the *Ros Airgead* had misread her position and was aground on the White Strand in Lough Kay, a mile further north. Kearney White's adventure of 1864 has already vividly recorded what can be expected in Lough Kay in bad weather. At 11 p.m. the lifeboat located the trawler aground on the sandy bottom of a dead lee shore. It was low water so the crew was out of danger, but it was impossible to get close enough to fire a line across.

At 1.30 a.m. the following morning, the lifeboat returned to Knightstown pier at Valentia and picked up a forty-gallon drum. On reaching the trawler she anchored and veered down the drum with sixty fathoms of line. The line was secured by the trawler's crew who passed a rope back to the lifeboat. Two hours later the trawler *Ros Muc* skippered by Mike 'Murt' O'Connell of Caherciveen also got a line fast aboard the *Ros Airgead*. The two boats failed to float the trawler. Coxswain O'Connell laid out two anchors to prevent the trawler drifting further into the shore. The lifeboat stood by until at low water the trawler was again out of danger.

The crew of the *Ros Airgead* came ashore and landed much of their gear and ballast and returned to their ship. The lifeboat returned to the casualty at 2 p.m. on the afternoon of the 27 November. At 6 p.m. that evening the *Ros Airgead* was towed clear by the lifeboat and the *Ros Muc*. For this service the thanks of the Institution inscribed on vellum was awarded to Coxswain Jeremiah O'Connell. A letter of appreciation was sent to Skipper Mike O'Connell of the *Ros Muc*.

The Rescue That Stank

Rescues are remembered for many reasons – violent storms, great seamanship or outstanding courage – but Valentia has one rescue that is remembered because it stank! The official report gives details of this rescue as follows:

At 11.48 on the night of 17th November 1955, a message was received from the Valentia Radio Station that the trawler 'Styvel' of Concarneau, France which had a crew of ten had wirelessed that she had broken down and was in distress near the Skelligs Rock. At 12.10 early on the 18th the lifeboat A.E.D, put out. The sea was moderate and there was a moderate south-easterly breeze and it was low water. The lifeboat made for the position and at 1.45 saw a rocket about seven miles South West of Bray Head. A little later she came up with the trawler half a mile North West of the Skelligs Rocks and went alongside. Ropes were passed across and the lifeboat towed the 'Styvel' to Valentia which was reached at 5.18. Just after they entered the harbour the 'Styvel', which had been holed on the Skelligs Rocks, sank a hundred yards from the pier head. The lifeboat rescued her crew and gave them hot drinks, and then landed them at 6.30. She put off again to warn the fishing fleet and finally reached her station at 10.00 o'clock. The French Ministry of the Merchant Navy expressed its thanks to the lifeboat crew.

But the story did not end there. The unforgettable stink arose some weeks later when a salvage company raised the vessel from the harbour bottom. The hold, which had been full of fish, now contained a stinking, decomposing mass. So vile was the stench that people passing along the seafront were known to become ill. Nobody could be found to enter the offensive hold until one local character,

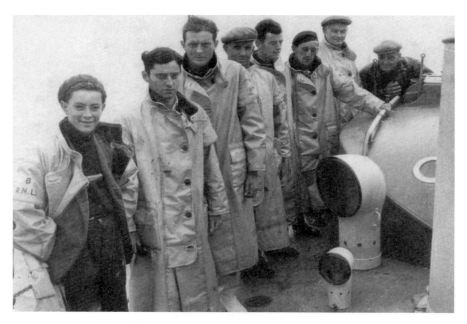

Valentia Lifeboat Crew, May 1956. From left to right: Johnny O'Connell R.I.P., James Lynch RIP, Des Lavelle, Johnny O'Shea RIP, Joseph Houlihan, John Shanahan, Jeremiah O'Connell RIP, John Dore RIP. Photo: Joseph Houlihan Collection.

making himself immortal by his proclamation, 'I see no smell, boy!', entered the hold, rolled up his sleeves and emptied it almost single handed.

After many weeks the salvage company had the engines repaired. The stem was repaired with plywood and the *Styvel* sailed for home, 'with a bone in her teeth'. The repairers had unfortunately underestimated the Atlantic swell. Hardly had she cleared the harbour mouth when the first big sea stripped the plywood from the vessel and she began to sink again. But she made it back to Knightstown under her own steam. The repairers got it right second time round and the *Styvel* eventually sailed safely to Concarneau, leaving pungent memories lingering in Valentia.

Rescue by Dingle Coast Lifesaving Service

At 11.40 p.m on the night of the 6 June 1956, the Dingle Coast Lifesaving Service telephoned that the fishing boat Carraig Doun, of Dublin, had engine trouble one mile west of Ventry harbour and was being driven ashore. Another trawler, *Elsie Mable*, was standing by to give the position to the lifeboat. At 12.12 the lifeboat *AED* put out in a very rough sea. A fresh westerly gale was blowing, and the tide was flooding. The lifeboat reached the position at 1.32 a.m. There were several other fishing boats in the area but contact could not be made by wireless. The lifeboat approached time and again to within fifty yards of the rocks, and using the searchlight, the coxswain made every effort to sight survivors or to locate the Carraig Doun, but without success. The fishing boat had used up all her flares, and it was clear that even if she had not been abandoned she would have been unable to indicate her position. There was now a west-south-westerly gale and heavy rain, and at times visibility was down to 100 yards. Seas were breaking over the lifeboat. At 5.32 a.m. the coxswain saw one survivor clinging to the rocks. He was unable to manoeuvre the lifeboat close in to effect a rescue, and it would have been unwise to use the breech's buoy. He therefore contacted the honorary secretary, asking for the information to be passed to the Coast Lifesaving Service at Dingle. This was done, and the Lifesaving Service rescued the man. All the fishing boats had by this time returned to harbour, and the lifeboat went to Dingle to find out how many men had been onboard the *Carraig Doun*. When it was known two men were missing, the lifeboat put out again with a local fisherman on board and carried out a further search, but she could find nothing. She then returned to her station, arriving back at 3.15 in the afternoon.

The *AED* remained at Valentia until September 1957. During her six-year term at Valentia she launched on service fifty-seven times and saved eighty-three lives. She was sold out of the service in 1957 and was last reported with a cabin added as a pleasure boat in Fuengirola in Spain in February 1992.

In 1956, Coxswain Jeremiah O'Connell and Assistant Mechanic Paddy Murphy visited a number of stations in the UK to advise on what would be a suitable lifeboat for Valentia. One boat they viewed was historical in so far as she was the first of the 47 foot Watson class. RNLB *Dunnett Head* (Civil Service No.31) was stationed at Thurso, northern Scotland. She was powered by twin Gardner sixty horse-power 5LW diesel engines, this being the first time that commercially built engines of this size were installed in an RNLI lifeboat. She also had a covered steering position, worm drive rather than the usual self centering. She was fitted with bulwarks fore and aft. This lifeboat had arrived in Thurso on 29 January 1956.

Shortly after their visit the Valentia men heard the news that, on 10 December of that year, the lifeboat and her slipway top boathouse were both destroyed by fire. In any event the boat that was chosen for Valentia was a Barnett class boat.

SEVEN

A NEW BARNETT CLASS LIFEBOAT –
ROWLAND WATTS

The Barnett class of lifeboat had been radically remodeled and in 1950 a new arrangement was accepted. The steering position was moved amidships and there was a wheelhouse and deck cabin. The first of the new generation of these boats to be stationed in Ireland was allocated to Valentia. Built at the yard of Groves and Guttridge in Cowes, Isle of Wight, the new boat RNLB *Rowland Watts* sailed from Cowes to Brixham, Newlyn, Ballycotton and arrived at Valentia 17 September 1957.

The *Rowland Watts*, funded by a legacy of Mr Rowland Watts of Colchester, Essex, cost £38,500. Her Official Number was 938. She was 52 feet in length,

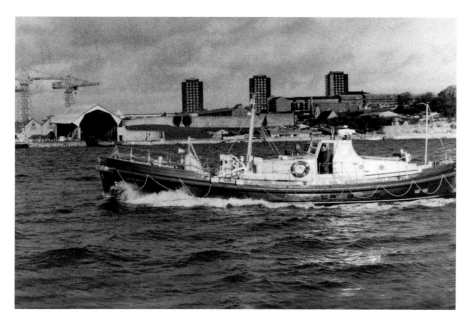

RNLB *Rowland Watts* in Plymouth after radar installation. Photo: Dermot Walsh Collection.

had a beam of 14 feet and a draft of 4 feet 7 inches. She was powered by two Gardner seventy-two horse-power diesel engines. She had a maximum speed of nine knots and a range of 254 miles at full speed. Her crew strength was eight and she could carry 100 survivors in bad weather.

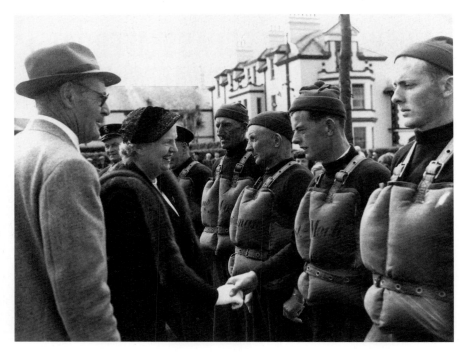

Above: Thursday 29 May 1958 at Knightstown pier. Mr Kieran O'Driscoll introduces the lifeboat crew to Mrs Sean T. O'Ceallaigh, wife of the President of Ireland before she formally named the lifeboat. From left to right: Coxswain J. O'Connell, Mechanic John Dore (partially obscured), Second Coxswain J. Sugrue, Bowman J. O'Shea, Assistant Mechanic J. Houlihan, Crewmember Des Lavelle. Photo: J & E Lavelle Collection.

Right: Mary Robinson presents flowers to Mrs Sean T. O'Ceallaigh. Photo: Dick Robinson Collection.

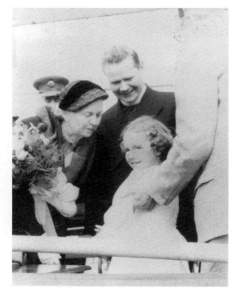

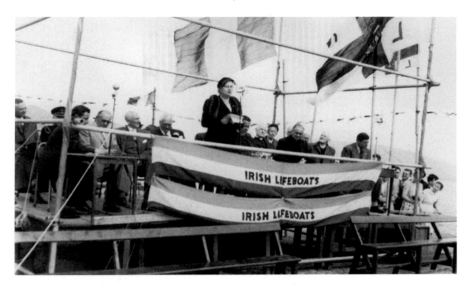

Mrs Sean T. O'Ceallaigh formally names the *Rowland Watts*. Photo: Dick Robinson Collection.

The Naming Ceremony

The official naming ceremony of the *Rowland Watts* was a day of great pomp and splendour. The 29 May 1958 was blessed with sunshine as dignitaries of Church and State were present at Knightstown pier. The village was radiant and bunting-bedecked. Ships in the harbour were dressed overall. Prior to the start of the ceremony a bouquet of flowers was presented to Mrs Sean T. O'Kelly, wife of the President of Ireland, by nine-year-old Mary Robinson of Knightstown. Most Revd Dr Denis Moynihan, Bishop of Kerry, blessed the lifeboat.

Mr Frank Watts formally presented the lifeboat, named after his uncle, whose bequest had paid for her, to the RNLI She was accepted by Captain the Honourable Valentine Wyndham Quinn, RN, Deputy Chairman of the RNLI In his speech he said, 'Valentia, where the boat has come to be stationed, is, you may be sure, very well known to the Committee of Management as a live and efficient station with a long record of good service.'

He praised the continuity of family service by Kieran O'Driscoll. Kieran O'Driscoll was recognized as one of the great characters of the lifeboat world, with many a story and anecdote on the subject. He took great pride in the fact that on one of the 'small' lifeboats the radio, which was supposed to have a ten-mile range, had picked up a radio station in Iceland. His most frequently told anecdote was of the terrier dog which chose to 'cock a leg' against the mortar from which a maroon was about to be fired. Upon the rocket zooming into the air and exploding, the poor mutt ran home screaming, in the door, up the stairs and took refuge under the bed.

Kieran would always swear by the 'Second Person of the Trinity' that, 'the bloody dog didn't piss for six months after that experience'. The honorary secretary, accepted the boat on behalf of the local station branch. Lieutenant Commander H.H. Harvey, Divisional Inspector of Lifeboats in Ireland, described the boat in all her detail. In her address Mrs O'Kelly said:

> The arrival of a new lifeboat at her station is always a great event to the people who live in and around the town or village from which the lifeboat puts out to the rescue. The naming ceremony is, therefore, a particularly happy event, and I think we can all take pride in the splendid boat it will shortly be my privilege to name. She is as fine a craft as money, ingenuity and skill can produce. We also know that she is in the very best of hands. Crews of Valentia Lifeboats have a splendid tradition of rescuing those in danger at sea, and I think many present today will recall the night of November 25th 1954, a night when a full gale was blowing from the north-west and the sea was extremely rough. On that night the trawler *Ros Airgead* went aground on the White Horse rocks. The Valentia crew, as always, was ready to answer the call at once. The conditions were such that they had to make four attempts to reach the lifeboat by the pulling boat before they could board her. It is in such conditions, when other craft are making for shelter or harbour that the lifeboats are called out to the rescue. The men who meet such challenges deserve our respect, our admiration and our gratitude, and in naming this splendid new lifeboat we should, I think, honour all those who are ready to put out in her. 'I have great pleasure in naming this splendid new lifeboat *Rowland Watts* – May God bless her and all who sail in her.

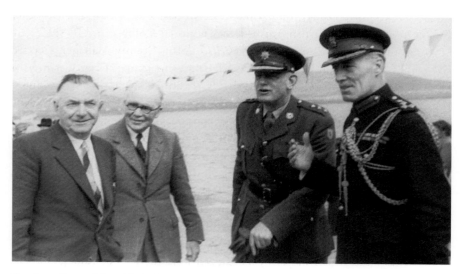

The Canadian and Spanish Ambassadors with Irish and British Army Officers. Photo: Dick Robinson Collection.

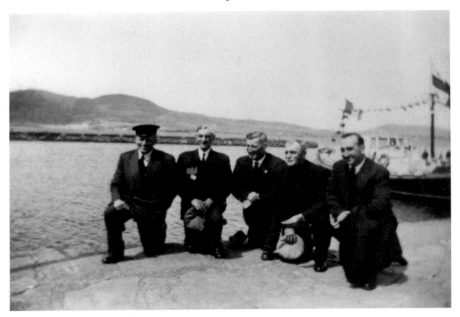

29 May 1958. Patsy Sliney, hero of Daunt Rock fame of 1936 (second left) and Richard Walsh of World Concord rescue fame in 1954 (centre) with coxwains from Kilmore Quay, Ballycotton and Kilronan at the *Rowland Watts* naming ceremony. Photo: Dick Robinson Collection.

Colonel R.J. Uniake DSO and Canon S.P. Howe MA, Rector of Valentia, also spoke. The ceremony was presided over by Revd T. O'Sullivan PP, chairman of the Valentia Branch. St Joseph's School Band from Tralee provided the music and hymns were sung by the local choir. The attendance included the Canadian Ambassador Mr Alfred Rive and Spanish Ambassador H.E. Mr Mariano de Yturralde Brigadier (who represented the British Ambassador), Colonel Collins Powell, Mrs H.M. Crowley. TD, Mr P.W. Palmer TD, Mr W.F. Quinlan, County Manager, Captain Kelly and Captain Kennedy of Irish Lights. Representatives of lifeboat stations at Helvick Head, Ballycotton, Courtmacsherry, Baltimore and Rosslare harbour as well as Captain Duggan of the Coast Lifesaving Service and Mr Tim O'Malley of Waterville Coast Lifesaving Service also attended. The legendary Ballycotton Coxswain Paddy Sliney, of Daunt Rock rescue fame, and Rosslare lifeboat hero Richard Walsh of the 'World Concord' rescue were amongst the guests.

The crew on the day were: Coxswain Jeremiah O'Connell, Second Coxswain Jack Sugrue, Mechanic John Dore, Assistant Mechanic Joseph Houlihan, Bowman John O'Shea, Seán Murphy, James Lynch, John Shanahan and Des Lavelle. The crew list at the time also included the Walsh Brothers, Paddy Murphy and Dan McCrohen.

The rating of bowman was really a hangover from the days of pulling and sailing lifeboats. So many were the hawsers and ropes associated with the anchor and securing the boat that one man was delegated to hold that position. In the

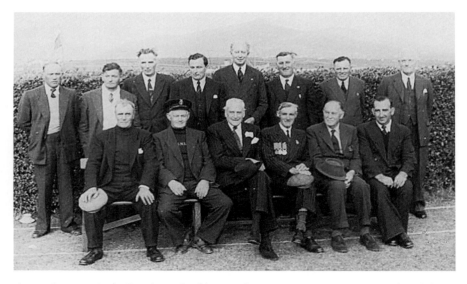

At a garden party in the Royal Hotel celebrating the naming ceremony. Front row, from left to right: -?-; Coxwain Jeremiah O'Connel, Captain the Honourable V.W. Wyndham Quinn, chairman of the RNLI; Ex-Coxwain Patrick Sliney (Gold medal holder of Daunt Rock rescue fame-Ballycotton); -?-; Coxswain Michael Lane-Walsh (Ballycotton). Back row: -?-; -?-; -?-; Lieutenant Commander H.H. Harvey, district inspector; Mr Frank Watts representing the donor; Coxswain Richard Walsh of Rosslare harbour (Silver Medal holder for World Concorde rescue); -?-. Photo: Dick Robinson Collection.

ordinary course the bowman would be next in line to the second coxswain to become coxswain. The position of bowman was phased out during the late 1970s and into the 1980s; the last bowman was at Skegness in Lincolnshire and relinquished the position in 1986.

The shore attendant was Ned Murphy. Members of the local committee present were H.H. Robinson Deputy Launching Authority and Officer-in-Charge at Valentia Radio, J.H. O'Neill, Batt Griffin NT, W. Shanahan, F.A. Whittlesey and W. McCrohen. After a short ceremonial cruise around the harbour the lifeboat returned to moorings. A garden party was held in the grounds of the Royal Hotel and a dance in St Derarcas' Hall rounded off the celebrations.

Maria on the Rocks at Portmagee

Six days later, on 4 June 1958, the new lifeboat answered her first service call, but it was by no means a classic rescue. The trawler *Maria*, registered in Waterford, but owned and fished from Portmagee, went aground on the Perch Rock in the Portmagee Channel, 800 yards from her home port. The lifeboat service consisted of standing by the casualty until the rising tide floated her off the rocks.

Maria in Trouble Again

Two weeks later the same *Maria* was the lifeboat's second customer in rather more difficult circumstances. This time she had engine trouble 25 miles north-west of Inis Tearaght some 40 miles from home in a north-westerly gale. The *Rowland Watts* saved the *Maria* and her crew of three without difficulty.

Jeremiah O'Connell retired from the position of coxswain on 31 October 1958. He had been twice awarded the thanks of the Institution inscribed on vellum. During his tenure of office, Valentia lifeboats launched on service ninety-five times and saved 101 lives. His successor was Jack Sugrue.

A Terrible Tragedy

The wreck of the *Marie Brigette* is a more significant event in the history of the *Rowland Watts*. This new 110-ton trawler from Concarneau in France broadcast a mayday distress call at 12.45 a.m. on the morning of Saturday 7 February 1959. This and a final message at 1.02 a.m. saying that the crew were abandoning ship 3 miles south of the Blaskets were received by Valentia Radio. Phone contact with lifeboat secretary Kieran O'Driscoll was finally made at 1.21 a.m. maroons were fired and the *Rowland Watts* was under way at 1.40 a.m. The lifeboat reached the search area at 3.10 a.m. and found nothing. Fenit lifeboat, a fleet of trawlers from Dingle, an Avro Shackleton aircraft from Ballykelly, an Irish Air Corps plane, the merchant ship *Manchester Spinner* and several French trawlers also joined the search. The first body was recovered at 9 a.m. by the French Trawler *Piccanninie*. By 10 a.m. Valentia lifeboat had recovered two bodies and some wreckage and now, with hindsight, it became clear that the position had been 3 miles south of Inistearaght and not 3 miles south of the Blaskets, and that the *Marie Brigette* had struck the Foze Rocks. After eleven hours of searching, and with a violently ill crewman, the *Rowland Watts* headed for Valentia with her somber cargo. It was now obvious that there were no survivors. Two French trawlers landed a further two bodies at Valentia. At an inquest held at Valentia, a principal officer from the Department of Posts and Telegraphs traced the history of the phone link with Valentia and the various arrangements and alternatives offered to the RNLI Valentia had but sixteen subscribers and twenty were needed for a full night service. A line was given to the No. 1 man on the Coast Lifesaving Service, and he could switch a call through to the honorary secretary. A notice on the switchboard at Caherciveen Exchange on the night of the emergency stating that the Valentia trunks were out of order had been so placed because the lines were noisy, not because they were out of order. The jury returned a verdict in accordance with the medical evidence that Desiree Furac (33), the Captain, Leon Fellin (52), Yves Ruric (53) and Francis Garrac (52) had died of exposure following immersion in the sea and that no blame attached to any one. The Coroner Dr Denis O'Donovan agreed with the verdict. He paid tribute to the lifeboat crews who launch in such conditions at great personal risk. The crew on this occasion were Coxswain Jack Sugrue, Mechanic John Dore, John Shanahan, Des Lavelle, Martin Connolly, Nealie O'Donovan, Eddie Murphy and Michael Murphy. By the time Valentia was joined to the direct dial system for national and international calls in November 1984 there were 110 phones on the island.

Life Boat Dragging Her Moorings

A hurricane raged from 13 to 15 November 1959. The *Rowland Watts* was seen to be dragging her anchor. She was being driven towards the 'Foot' (the sandbar that runs out into the harbour from the breakwater pier). The crew was put on board by the ferryboat and the lifeboat was taken to moorings in the shelter of Beginish Island, where she spent the night. She returned to Knightstown Quay the following day. On the Sunday morning, with extra hands, moorings were re-laid in an operation taking seven hours.

Fishing Boat Broken Down

On 9 March 1960, Valentia Radio received a message 'Fishing Vessel Ross Corr position: mouth of Ballinskelligs Bay requires urgent assistance, drifting with broken engine.' The lifeboat *Peter and Sarah Blake* put to sea. At 7.45 p.m. she found the trawler drifting 3 miles south of Bolus Head, near Scarriff Island in a heavy swell in a south-easterly force six wind. The trawler was taken in tow to Portmagee. During the passage to the casualty the fact that the service occurred on Ash Wednesday gave rise to debate on board the lifeboat. The soup supplied to the lifeboats was mock turtle soup. But was it meat or fish? One could not eat meat on Ash Wednesday. I fail to remember the result of the debate. It was my first time on service on the boat. I ate the soup with relish as my belly was almost stuck to my backbone with the cold.

Propeller Lost

At 2.55 p.m. on the afternoon of the 5 September 1960, a mayday message was received from Valentia radio station that the fishing vessel *Ros Ceaion* was adrift in Blasket Sound and needed help. There was a moderate south-westerly wind with a corresponding sea, and the tide was flooding. At 3.05 p.m. the lifeboat *Rowland Watts* was launched. She found the *Ros Ceaion* close to the rocks at Inish Nabro. The fishing vessel had lost her propeller and was in extreme danger.

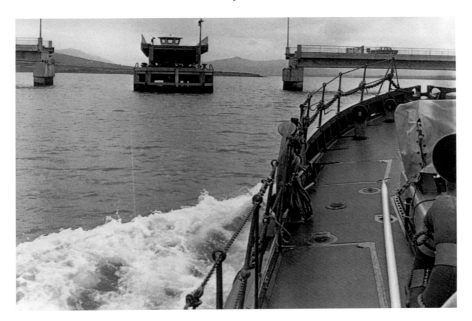

The *Rowland Watts* about to pass through the bridge. Photo: Dick Robinson Collection.

The lifeboat took her in tow. Because of the severe swell the tow parted but was re-secured using the wire from the winch. The trawler was berthed at Portmagee. The lifeboat then returned to her station, arriving at 1.45 a.m. on 6 September. Because of the weather conditions all the fishing vessel's gear had to be abandoned.

Body Recovered

On 9 September 1960 J. O'Donnell, a van driver from Killorglin, was asked by a party of bathers to contact the lifeboat. One of their number was missing. The *Rowland Watts* lifeboat recovered the body of Lieutenant Colonel John Marshall. Artificial respiration was applied and continued until the lifeboat reached Valentia Quay. At the request of the coroner the following letter was sent to the Secretary of the RNLI at 42 Grosvenor Gardens, London:

Dear Sir,
At an inquest held on the 9th September, a verdict of accidental death due to drowning was returned on Lieut-Col John Marshall, 71 Granmore Lane, Aldershot. The Coroner asked that the following be conveyed to the Lifeboat Institution. 'The speed and efficient manner in which the lifeboat was launched

and the excellent way in which the crew carried out their duty, reflects the highest possible credit.'

During his evidence Coxswain J. Sugrue stated that the lifeboat was awash and that the Crewmen had great difficulty recovering the body.

Yours faithfully,

Kieran O' Driscoll.

Honorary Secretary.

Trawler Located in Fog

On the 16 December 1960, the local trawler *Ros Airgead* was adrift about 5 miles west of Bray Head. The lifeboat *Peter and Sarah Blake* was launched at 8.30 a.m. In a fine feat of seamanship by Second Coxswain John Shanahan, the trawler was located and taken in tow to Valentia. During the tow the fog was so dense that the casualty was not visible from the lifeboat.

Fishing Vessel with Fouled Propeller

Three days later, on the 19 December 1960, the *Ros Airgead* was again in difficulty. She had a wire rope on her propeller and was ten mile north-west of Valentia. The *Peter and Sarah Blake* was launched, again under Second Coxswain John Shanahan at 3.30 p.m.

The wind was northerly force eight and the seas were rough and the tide in flood. It was bitterly cold with snow showers. Because of the weather conditions it was decided to enter the harbour via the Portmagee entrance. The tow parted three times and was reconnected. The local committee recommended an extra award to Second Coxswain Shanahan for this service.

Surgical Team Conveyed to Island

On 26 February 1961, the services of the lifeboat were requested. A surgical team led by the County Surgeon (Mr Galvin) was travelling from Tralee to carry out an emergency operation at the local cottage hospital.

There was a south-west gale and a flood tide. The *Peter and Sarah Blake* collected the team and conveyed them to the island from Caherciveen pier. The lifeboat stood by until 4.15 p.m. when the team was returned to Caherciveen. A number of people who had been weather bound on the mainland were brought back to Valentia.

French Crew Came Ashore Safely

On 5 December 1961, a French Trawler the *Piense Paysane* was wrecked off Ballydavid Head. Eight men were believed adrift in a rubber dingy. The *Rowland Watts* sailed at 9.50 a.m. and arrived in the search area at 11.40 a.m. The seas were rough in a north-westerly force six and a flood tide. There were snow and hail showers and it was bitterly cold. The missing men came ashore in a small cove known as Cuas. The lifeboat was recalled and returned to station at 3.15 p.m.

Injured Light Keeper Landed

On 1 July 1961, the honorary secretary received the following message from the Inis Tearaght Lighthouse, 'Badly injured man on rock, requires lifeboat and doctor as soon as possible. Man's head badly cut and back injury'. The *Peter and Sarah Blake* lifeboat was brought to Knightstown Quay. The doctor was embarked and with the boarding boat in tow the lifeboat went to the Tearaght. The landing was awash. The doctor was landed by hoist from the boarding boat. The casualty was placed in the lifeboat stretcher. The stretcher was brought down the 300 steps. It was swung out on the hoist and lowered to the boarding boat and conveyed to the lifeboat. The boarding boat returned and the doctor was lowered on the hoist and returned to the lifeboat. There was a heavy swell and a force five north-

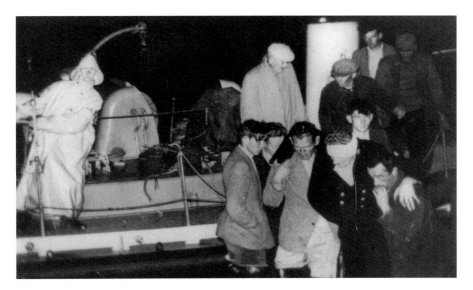

12.30 a.m. on 2 July 1961. Injured lighthouse keeper Patrick O'Shea is assisted ashore from the relief lifeboat *Peter and Sarah Blake* by Dermot Walsh and Eddie Murphy. Dr P. McKenna (white cap) accompanied the crew and rendered medical aid. Photo: courtesy of Des Lavelle.

easterly wind during the operation. The casualty was landed at Renard point. He was conveyed to Tralee General Hospital and made a full recovery.

Teenagers Adrift in Yawl

On 31 August 1962, a message was received from Mr E. O'Mahony, chairman, Caherciveen Lifesaving that six children were adrift in a yawl under oars and half a mile from Cuascrom pier in Dingle Bay. The *Peter and Sarah Blake* relief lifeboat sailed at 5.10 p.m. and contacted the yawl at 5.50 p.m. The yawl was at the harbour entrance and was escorted in by the lifeboat. The parents of the children telephoned the honorary secretary to express their thanks and congratulation on the speed with which the call was answered. They informed the honorary secretary that the boat had been taken without the owners permission and that only one boy knew how to row. There were four girls and two boys in the boat.

Casualty and Towing Vessel Escorted In

On 17 October 1962, the fishing vessel *Pride of Ballinskelligs* was reported overdue. There were two people on board. The lifeboat *Rowland Watts* slipped moorings at 10.52 p.m. Four miles north-west of Valentia Lighthouse the casualty was picked up by searchlight. As the fishing vessel *Ros Airgead* was within half a mile of the boat they took her in tow to Caherciveen. The lifeboat escorted both vessels into Valentia harbour and returned to moorings.

Ill Man Taken off Skelligs

On 16 June 1963, the relief lifeboat *Mary Stanford* slipped her moorings at 1.50 p.m. She was launched in response to a request to bring an ill man from the Skelligs Lighthouse. With a relief keeper on board and the boarding boat in tow the lifeboat reached the Skelligs at 3.50 p.m. The sick man was landed at 6.30 p.m. where he was attended to by Dr O'Donoghue and removed to hospital.

Diver Lost

On 19 June 1963, the *Rowland Watts* was involved in a search for a diver off Doulous Head. Four local boats joined the search, together with members of the local sub-aqua club. The body of James Hewitt of Gateshead Co. Durham was recovered in 80 feet of water by local diver Des Lavelle. At an inquest the following day the verdict was that death was due to asphyxia due to drowning. John Butler of the Office of Public Works stated that he had seen the dead man's diving equipment and it appeared to be in perfect condition.

Casualty Reached Shore Safely

On 30 July 1963, the *Rowland Watts* was launched at 11.45 p.m. to search for three visitors missing in a 14 foot fibre glass dingy with an outboard motor. They were last reported 1½ miles west of Kells Bay. The wind was south-easterly force six in a moderate sea and visibility was poor.

At 12.40 a.m. a message was received from Michael Grimes of Cork, one of the missing men. 'Please thank all concerned. Our motor had broken down and we landed at Flesk Cove and returned on foot along the mountain. We could not row against the gale. We can see the searchlight of the lifeboat outside the cove where we left the dingy.' The lifeboat was immediately recalled.

Ill Man Taken from Ship

On 21 December 1963 the *Rowland Watts* launched at 2.10 a.m. She embarked a doctor and a nurse and put to sea to make rendezvous with the 6,000-ton *Wellpark* of Glasgow. One of the crew had acute appendicitis. He was taken on board the lifeboat 5 miles west of the Skelligs and landed at Renard quay at 7.30 a.m. where an ambulance was waiting to take him to the County Hospital in Tralee.

Ill Woman Landed at Mainland

On 12 May 1964 the *Rowland Watts* was launched at 1.15 a.m. to convey a very ill female patient to Renard Point. The patient and a nurse were embarked. The lifeboat had to stand off at the pier due to the weather and the state of the tide. When a window of opportunity presented itself the patient was landed into the care of the waiting ambulance team. The lifeboat returned to station at 3 a.m.

Escort for Spanish Vessels

On 26 June 1964 the *Rowland Watts* launched at 9.45 p.m. to go to the assistance of the Spanish fishing vessel *Vispon* of La Corunna. Her engine room was flooding and she was reported to be 9 miles west of the Bull Rock. In thick fog she was found at 2.29 a.m. in tow of another Spanish trawler *Muella*. The lifeboat

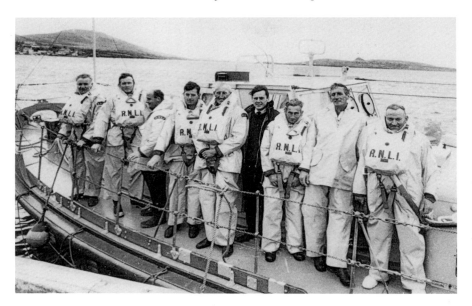

Ted Cahill, Des Lavelle, Tony O Connor, Joe Houlihan, Jack Sugrue, Kevin Devane, Paddy Murphy, Dermot Walsh, Miko Leary. Photo: courtesy of the RNLI.

was requested to escort both vessels to Bantry. The lifeboat and the two trawlers arrived at Bantry at 1.50 p.m. on 27 June. The *Vispon's* deck was awash when she was moored to Bantry Quay.

Body of Electrician Landed

On 4 December 1964, the *Rowland Watts* responded to a call from the German vessel *Waldemar Peter*. She requested the lifeboat to meet her, with a doctor on board in Dingle Bay. The lifeboat was alongside the ship at 11.15 p.m. Ten miles north-west of Valentia. The casualty, the electrician Johannes Schaale, was transferred to the lifeboat. He died at 11.35 p.m. while on passage to Valentia. As the doctor was on board a death certificate could be issued without the need for an inquest. The man died of cardiac failure. The body was landed at Valentia. Arrangements were made with the German Embassy to have the body sent to Hamburg.

Revellin of Spain Saved

On 14 April 1965, the honorary secretary received the following message from Valentia Radio, 'There is a Spanish Fishing Vessel sending out mayday call, position not given but strength of signals would indicate the vessel close to Valentia.

We are trying to get Caherciveen 26 to answer the telephone and act as inter- preter.' The lifeboat *Mary Stanford*, on temporary duty at Valentia, launched at 5 a.m. At 5.45 a.m Valentia Radio gave the position of the casualty, the fishing boat *Revellin* of Spain with fourteen crew, as approximately 51.56 north 10.23 west. The lifeboat found the casualty at 6.30 a.m. She was riding at anchor and was being driven towards the shore. The wind was north-west force five to six the sea rough and the weather was bad. At the request of the master a tow line was passed and towing proceeded towards Valentia. The tow parted at 8 a.m. A wire hawser for the casualty was passed across and she was towed safely to Valentia.

Doctor Taken to German Ship

On the 14 October 1965 the *MV Ginnheim* of Bremen, Germany sent out a message seeking urgent medical assistance. Passenger vessels close to her offered assistance but in adverse conditions could not transfer a doctor. Arrangements were made for the Valentia lifeboat to meet her when she closed the Irish Coast.

The rendezvous was fixed for a position 5 miles north of Bray Head at 10 a.m. on 16 October. The *Rowland Watts* slipped moorings at 9 a.m. She proceeded to sea with Dr Healy, who offered his services in the absence of the Honorary Medical Adviser, and a television camera man onboard. The sea was rough. There was a force six east-north-easterly wind and showers. On reaching the vessel, Coxswain Sugrue positioned the lifeboat on the starboard side of the vessel. Given the conditions, he asked the ship to proceed another 3 miles into the bay. Here, with fenders on the port side and Second Coxswain D. Walsh in charge of deck operations, the doctor was put onto the ladder on the top of a large wave by Second Coxswain Walsh assisted by crew member Des Lavelle. The crew member was treated on board the ship. The patient did not need to be transferred. The conditions ruled out the doctor using the ladder. With the aid of some of the crew of the Ginnheim and on instructions of the lifeboat crew the doctor jumped. He was caught by members of the lifeboat crew. He and the television cameraman were landed at Valentia.

Kieran O'Driscoll resigned as honorary secretary on the 25 August 1967. Tributes were paid to Kieran O'Driscoll on his retirement. Mr H. Robinson and Kevin Devane were appointed joint honorary secretaries. Mr Robinson left the island in September 1968 on his retirement as officer-in-charge at Valentia Radio. Kevin Devane was appointed honorary secretary. On the 11 November 1968, Kevin Devane vacated the position of honorary secretary. P.J. Gallagher and Johnny Reidy were appointed joint honorary secretaries. This arrangement was changed on the 18 November. Mr Gallagher was appointed honorary secretary and Mr Reidy was appointed assistant honorary secretary and deputy launching authority. In 1971, Tim Lyne and Ian Bardon were appointed deputy launching authorities.

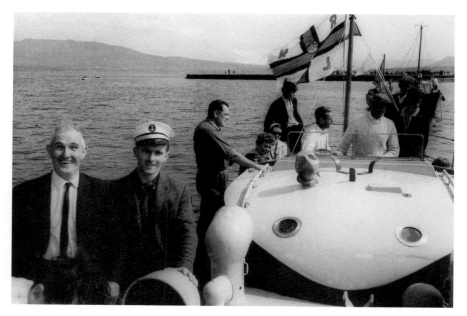

Regatta Day, August 1968. The lifeboat leaving the moorings. From left to right: Joe Robinson, honorary secretary; Dick Robinson, crew; -?-; Small Paddy Murphy, second mechanic; Jack Sugrue, coxswain; -?-. Photo: Dick Robinson Collection.

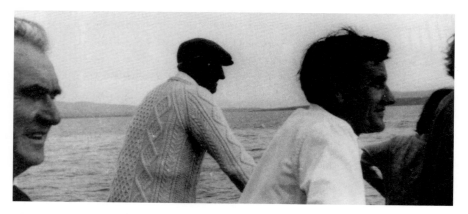

The honorary secretary has a go! 'Joe' Robinson takes a turn at the wheel of the relief lifeboat *Peter and Sarah Blake*, August 1968. Coxswain Jack Sugrue is in the centre and his son John right. John was awarded a long-service badge at Howth. Photo: Dick Robinson Collection.

Man Landed from Inis Tearaght

On 23 March 1968, Captain Harrison of Irish Lights contacted the honorary secretary and asked if the lifeboat could take a tradesman ashore from Inis Tearaght lighthouse. The man's mother had died. The lighthouse was contacted and a relief was not possible on that day. It was arranged that when conditions were suitable the lighthouse keepers would contact the lifeboat coxswain. At 7.27 a.m. on 24 March the coxswain was told that a landing was possible. The *Rowland Watts* slipped her moorings at 8 a.m. and proceeded to sea with the boarding boat in tow. The lighthouse informed the lifeboat that landing on the South Landing was not possible. They could use their own judgment on the North Landing. After inspecting the North Landing it was deemed not possible to effect a relief and the lifeboat returned to station.

Fishing Vessel Broken Down

On 17 July 1968 Valentia Radio informed the honorary secretary at 4.07 p.m. that the fishing vessel *Lios Dairbhre* was broken down one mile east of Doulous Head and needed lifeboat assistance. As the crew were already near at hand the lifeboat *Peter and Sarah Blake* launched with the Second Coxswain Dermot Walsh in command. They reached the casualty at 5 p.m. and took her in tow to Valentia.

Sick Man Taken from Lighthouse

On 30 July 1968, Captain Harrison of Irish Lights requested that the lifeboat bring a sick man ashore from Inis Tearaght Lighthouse. The lifeboat *Peter and Sarah Blake* slipped moorings at 3.12 p.m. and with the boarding boat in tow proceeded at best speed to the lighthouse. Second Coxswain Dermot Walsh was in command. The weather was good with a choppy sea. At 5.39 p.m the lifeboat had embarked the patient and he was landed at Valentia at 7.36 p.m.

Tragedy that put Lifeboat Crew at Extreme Personal Risk

In terms of 'great personal risk' the night of the *Seaflower* disaster is regarded in Valentia as one of the most terrible nights that the lifeboat experienced. This trawler from Castletownbere was in difficulties on rocks at the entrance to Ardgroom harbour on the southern side of Kenmare River. Valentia Radio received word of the distress at 1.21 a.m. on the morning of Sunday 22 December 1968 and the *Rowland Watts* set out at 1.35 a.m. into a south-westerly hurricane on her thirty-three-mile journey to Ardgroom. Dermot Walsh, then second coxswain, remains convinced that on this service, on at least one occasion, the *Rowland Watts* heeled over beyond 120 degrees, and should by all mathematical calculations have capsized. Indeed if ever a lifeboat crew were in peril the Valentia crew were on that night. Giant seas, driven by a hurricane, crashing against high cliffs and sending a backwash to come in conflict with the next onslaught of huge seas, the tide in the third hour of flood and the wind in another direction provided the recipe for maelstrom and mayhem. Other men of great courage had put to sea as well.

The *Ard Beara*, from nearby Castletownbere, also answered the call and put to sea in conditions for which she most certainly had not been built. At 3.35 a.m. the *Ard Beara* warned the lifeboat that the rocks close to the casualty were awash and at 5.15 a.m. she reported that the lights of the *Seaflower* had disappeared. The lifeboat at this time was still about 10 miles from Ardgroom. On her arrival in the dangerous and treacherous search area the lifeboat lit the area with parachute flares and assisted by the *Ard Beara* carried out a comprehensive search. At daylight, with a hurricane still blowing and dreadful seas lashing even the innermost reaches of Kenmare River, both boats picked up wreckage and life-jackets. At 2.40 p.m. two bodies in life jackets were reported off Ardea Castle; the lifeboat combed the area but nothing was found. Valentia Radio informed the lifeboat at 6.05 p.m. that the bodies of all five crew members of the *Seaflower* had been found by the Gardaí. The sad search was over.

As with every disaster there was much comment in the press. Two matters were beyond dispute. Had somebody competent seen and acted upon distress signs which, with hindsight, were noticeable for some hours before the alarm was raised, then this tragic loss of life may have been averted. Coxswain Sugrue and the Valentia lifeboat crew turned out extremely quickly and made a gallant attempt to save these five lives. At a meeting of the Committee of Management of

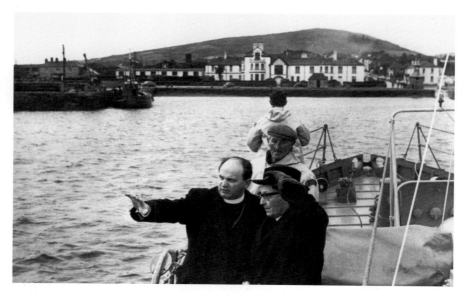

Dr Eamonn Casey, Bishop of Kerry with P.P. Fr Beasley and Ex-Coxswain Jack Sugrue.
Photo: courtesy of the *Kerryman*.

the RNLI on 13 March 1969 it was resolved that a letter of thanks, signed by the Secretary, be sent to the coxswain and crew in recognition of their services on the occasion. The coroner at the inquest referred to the lack of a Coastguard service, but the lesson terminated there.

Jack Sugrue was to retire from the position of Coxswain in 1969, but it would be no gentle winding down. The run up to his retirement was to be the year in which Valentia lifeboat saved the greatest number of lives in any year of its history to that point. There were thirteen services in that year and forty-five lives were saved. Non-lifesaving or effective services were on 4 and 29 June, and 1, 13, and 26 July and 3 August. The effective services were as follows:

23 January 1969 – MV *Thelka* of Norway

Saved boat and rescued fourteen.
Mr J. Reidy, assistant honorary secretary, received a call from Valentia Radio at 3.16 p.m. that fourteen persons on board the German ship *Thelka* needed assistance. In a rough sea and a force seven southerly wind the *Rowland Watts* slipped moorings at 3.34 p.m. and came up with the casualty 2 miles north of Doulous Head at 4.05 p.m. The vessel had no proper engine power or steering. She could only make two knots and could not progress against the gale. She was taken in tow to Valentia harbour. As Dermot Walsh, second coxswain and Des Lavelle crewman were away from the island John Curtin and John Reidy were called on as crewmen.

11 June 1969 – MFV *Ros Molt*

Saved boat and rescued five.
At 10.40 a.m. Valentia Radio informed the assistant honorary secretary, that the trawler *Ros Mult* was drifting off Loop Head Co. Clare. The *Rowland Watts* slipped her moorings at 10.50 a.m. She reached the casualty at 4.15 p.m. and took her in tow to Dingle. The lifeboat returned to station at 1.15 a.m. on 12 June. This was the first service into what was heretofore the Fenit Lifeboat territory. That boat had recently been withdrawn.

22 June 1969 – MFV *Siveen*

Saved boat and rescued five.
At 3.55 p.m. the honorary secretary was informed by Valentia Radio that the fishing vessel *Siveen* with five people on board required urgent assistance. She was off Beenacry Head and had a rope fouled on her propeller. She was anchored

by the propellor. The *Rowland Watts* slipped moorings at 4.05 p.m. The *Peter and Sarah Blake* lifeboat was coming from Baltimore to Valentia and also responded to the emergency call. With the aid of the two lifeboats the rope was cut and the *Rowland Watts* took the *Siveen* in tow to Caherciveen pier.

23 June 1969 – MFV *Eilis*

Saved boat and rescued four.
On 23 June 1969, at 12.25 p.m. the honorary secretary picked up a message from Valentia Radio stating that the fishing vessel *Eilis* had lost her rudder near Inistearaght in the Blaskets group of Islands. The *Peter and Sarah Blake* slipped moorings in a moderate sea and force five north-westerly wind. The *Eilis* was taken in tow at 3.25 p.m. and brought safely to Valentia at 6.05 p.m.

25 June 1969 - MFV *Kells Bay*

Saved boat and rescued four.
At 5.50 p.m. on 25 June 1969 in rough seas and a force six south-westerly wind, Dr Michael Grimes of Kells requested assistance. The boat was *Kells Bay*, with a boat man and three English anglers on board. The *Peter and Sarah Blake* proceeded to Foilage Point. There they took the boatman and anglers, who were wet and fatigued, on board. They were given hot soup. The *Kells Bay* was taken in tow to Kells pier where the survivors were landed and the boat secured. As coxswain Jack Sugrue was gone to Baltimore with the *Rowland Watts* Seán Murphy was in command of the lifeboat. Seán was skipper of the *Eilis* which had been rescued on 23 June.

1 July 1969 – MFV *Lios Dairbhre*

Gave help.
The Peter and Sarah Blake was launched at 4.05 p.m. in response to a call for assistance from the *Lios Dairbhre*. The lifeboat found her in tow of another vessel and returned to station.

Archbishop Adrift

On 13 July at 11.10 a.m. the honorary secretary was informed that the vessel *Skellig Michael* had not reached Dingle having set out from Caherciveen. There were fourteen people on board. At 11.15 a.m. the Gardaí at Dingle reported that a vessel appeared to be drifting off the entrance to Dingle harbour. In thick fog the *Peter and Sarah Blake* was launched at 11.30 a.m. and proceeded to the search area. At 11.45 a.m. a message was received that the *Skellig Michael* had arrived at Dingle. One of the passengers on the casualty was Most Revd Dr Morris Archbishop of Cashel and Emly.

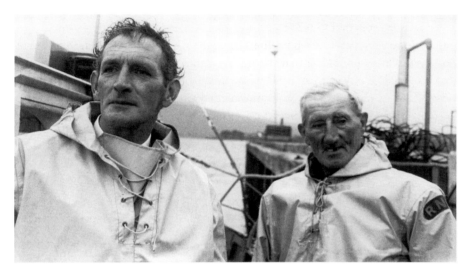

Dermot Walsh (coxswain) and Jack Sugrue (retired coxswain). Photo: courtesy of the RNLI.

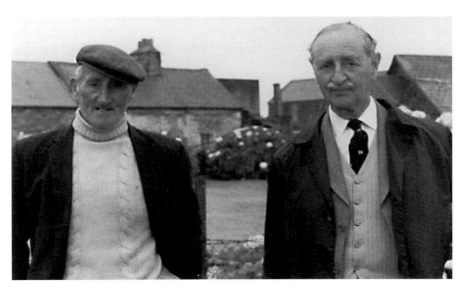

Ex-Coxswain Jack Sugrue with Major General Ralph Farrant, chairman of RNLI Committee of Management. Photo: courtesy of the RNLI.

20 July 1969

Twelve people stranded on Great Blasket Island – saved twelve.

This was an interesting service. On the 15 July a party of ornithologists, zoologists and a television crew were landed on the Great Blasket Island. They were to stay twenty-four hours and had supplies appropriate to that stay. The boat that was to collect them failed to return. Eventually after five days the tanker *Point Law* saw people waving what looked like white flags (it transpired that they were babies' nappies), and reported to Valentia Radio. RNLB *Peter and Sarah Blake* launched under Coxswain Sugrue, with two extra crew and the boarding boat in tow. In choppy seas and force four to five north-westerly winds the boarding boat with four crew and Second Coxswain Dermot Walsh in charge made several trips. All the people and their equipment being brought on board the lifeboat. Wet, cold and exhausted the rescued were given soup, corned beef, biscuits, some rum and cigarettes. The most vulnerable, a four-month-old baby boy, was fortunately being nursed by his mother and survived his ordeal.

A Rescue off Loop Head

The service to the *Ros Molt* was simple in lifeboating terms. The distress message was received at 10.40 a.m. The lifeboat slipped her moorings at 10.50 a.m., came up with the trawler at Loop Head at 4.15 p.m., took her in tow to Dingle and returned to station at 1.15 a.m. on 12 June 1969. This was the first service in what had heretofore been the bailiewick of the Fenit lifeboat. On the occasion of his retirement Jack Sugrue told *The Kerryman*, 'They were great years. I like to think that during my time with the service we did a lot of good. I am enjoying my retirement, but a little bit of me will always be at sea with the lifeboat'. Declining an offer to stay longer at the helm, he felt that the time had come to hand over to a younger man. That man was Dermot Walsh, who would soon be involved in the *Oranmore* rescue with the consequent award of a Silver Medal.

Fire Seen on Great Blasket

The first launch of the *Rowland Watts* with Dermot Walsh as coxswain came on 9 October 1969. The Gardaí at Ballyferriter reported that fires had been seen on the Great Blasket Island the night before. They were aware that a writer had been on the island for some time. No delivery of food to him had taken place for three weeks due to bad weather. The lifeboat slipped moorings at 9.14 a.m. and set out with the boarding boat in tow. Reaching the island at 10.45 a.m. and calling on the loud hailer, Coxswain Walsh sent the boarding boat with a crew of four to the island. The man was taken on board the lifeboat and returned to station at 1.45 p.m.

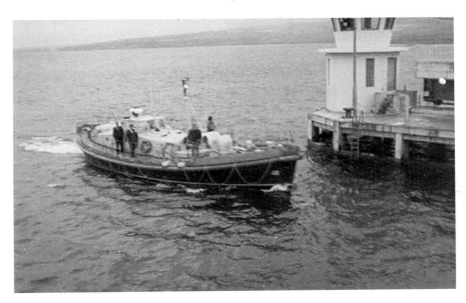

Above and below: August 1974 entering and exiting the openings span of Valentia Bridge.
Photos: Dick Robinson.

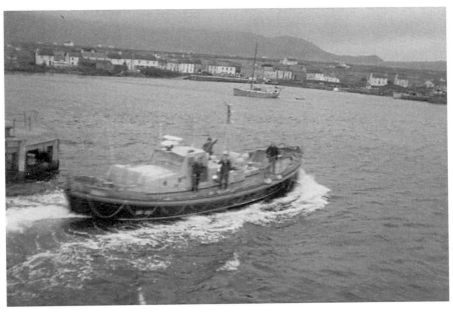

Response to Red Flares

At 9.55 p.m. on 22 October 1969 the Dingle trawler reported seeing red flares 2 miles north-west of Bray Head. The *Rowland Watts* was launched. At 10.25 p.m. the *Ard Fionbarr* reported flares south of her.

The *Nicholas Ann* also reported seeing flares and was proceeding to give aid. At 10.35 p.m. the *Rowland Watts* came up with the trawler *Granat* with a crew of five. Her propeller was fouled. The lifeboat took her in tow to Valentia. It transpired that the *Granat* had no radio in operation.

Passenger Boat Overdue

At 5.55 p.m on 23 May 1970 the honorary secretary was informed by Dr Holder, managing director of Irish Helicopters Ltd, that a boat *Brid* had left the Skelligs Rock with twenty-two people on board. She had not arrived at Portmagee. The helicopter company had been conveying people to the rock. After a number had been landed the helicopter was grounded the people had to be brought back by boat.

The lifeboat *Peter and Sarah Blake* was launched at 6.15 p.m. with the Second Coxswain Des Lavelle in command. At 7.15 p.m. the honorary secretary informed the lifeboat that the *Brid* had arrived at Portmagee. As the evening was getting blustery and the distance to the Skelligs is 9 miles of rough sea area, a request from Dr Michael Grimes of Kerry Boats Ltd that the lifeboat bring ashore fifteen people from the Skelligs was granted. At 7.40 p.m. Acting Coxswain Lavelle reported that all fifteen people had been embarked and returned to station.

The honorary secretary remarked, 'Coxswain D. Walsh was not available for this service so Second Coxswain D. Lavelle Took command of ON 755. Second Coxswain Lavelle and the crew did an excellent job of work and carried out their duties in an efficient manner.'

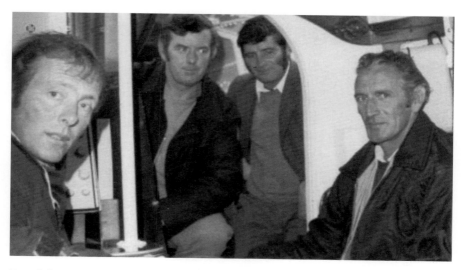

From left to right: Des Lavelle, second coxswain; Joe Houlihan, mechanic; Jimmy Murphy, second mechanic; Dermot Walsh, coxswain. Photo: Courtesy of the RNLI.

Fishing Boat Overdue

On 6 June 1970 the honorary secretary received a report that the angling boat *Siveen* was overdue. The *Peter and Sarah Blake* slipped moorings at 11.30 p.m. and proceeded to the Bray Head Area where the vessel had last been reported. After a search of the Bray Head area involving the use of parachute flares the casualty was eventually located 9 miles south-south-west of Bray Head. The casualty, with three people on board, was taken in tow to Caherciveen pier. The transmitter on the *Siveen* was out of order. The lifeboat was back at her moorings at 6.30 a.m. on 7 June.

Divers Reported Overdue

At 11.15 p.m. on 7 June the lifeboat *Peter and Sarah Blake* slipped moorings again with the cutter in tow. This followed a report from the Ballyferriter Gardaíthat that two skin divers who left Dunquin for the Blaskets at 9.30 a.m. had not returned. Their wives had contacted the Gardaí, who also reported a red flare fired from the Great Blasket. On reaching the Blasket Sound people were heard calling and the cutter went ashore. There were four skin divers there. They mentioned firing a white flare and said that their dingy and engine became submerged and they came ashore on the island. Two men were taken on board the lifeboat by the Cutter. They were cold and hungry and were given food and rum by the coxswain. They were landed at Valentia.

Search in Dense Fog; Sick Light Keeper Landed (Two Services in a Day)

On 27 August 1970 the *Peter and Sarah Blake* launched at 11 p.m., with Second Coxswain Des Lavelle in command, Coxswain D. Walsh being ill. A lobster boat was reported missing in Ballinskelligs Bay by Captain T. O'Malley of Waterville Coast Lifesaving Service. In dense fog, visibility being fifteen yards from the time the lifeboat passed the Wireless Point, the lifeboat searched from the Bolus Head area for six hours. The Gardaí at Waterville reported that the two men had come ashore. The lifeboat returned to Valentia.

On reaching Valentia Acting Coxswain Lavelle was informed that a relief light-house keeper needed to be brought to Inis Tearaght lighthouse and an injured keeper brought ashore. After refueling, the *Peter and Sarah Blake* set out with the boarding boat in tow. She reached the lighthouse at 8.20 p.m. and at 9.30 p.m. with the injured keeper on board she returned to Valentia at full speed. The crew came ashore at 12.45 p.m. on 29 August after a long day.

Trawler on Fire

On 17 November 1970 the Spanish trawler *Mero of Vigo* was reported on fire by a Shakleton aircraft. The lifeboat *Peter and Sarah Blake* slipped her moorings at 2.30 p.m. with Seán Murphy (skipper of the trawler *Eilis* in command). At 5.10 p.m. Valentia reported to the lifeboat that the survivors had been picked up and she changed course to return to station.

At 5.40 p.m. Shackelton aircraft *Playmate 16* reported that the survivors were still in the sea and the lifeboat headed back for the casualty area. On arrival the lifeboat found that all fourteen men had been picked up by the Spanish trawler *Mirabel*. The lifeboat returned to station. Spanish trawlers in the area had caused great confusion by reporting that they had picked up the survivors a long time before they were actually rescued.

Two People Rescued

At 3.30 a.m. on 1 August 1971 the Gardaí at Caherciveen reported that two men had taken a dingy from Valentia and gone towards Cromwell's Point Lighthouse. The *Rowland Watts* lifeboat slipped moorings at 3.50 a.m. At that time cries for help were heard in the distance. The coxswain fired a parachute flare. The casualty was seen about 400 yards from the moorings. The searchlight was turned on and the two people were rescued. Alan Glanville, who had raised the alarm, reported at the lifeboat house that his two friends were very drunk when they took the boat without permission.

Tug Escorted

In rough seas on 31 August 1971 the tug *Gnat* fired red flares off Rossbeigh Strand. The *Rowland Watts* slipped moorings at 1.30 p.m. At 3.50 p.m. the master reported that they had repaired the engine but asked the lifeboat to escort them to Castlemaine harbour, which they did.

Service to Fishing Vessel in Bad Weather

On 25 September 1971 the trawler *St Colette* requested lifeboat assistance. She was north of the Foze Rock. The *Peter and Sarah Blake*, with Second Coxswain Des Lavelle in charge slipped moorings at 3.15 p.m. The weather was bad with very bad visibility, a rough sea and south-westerly wind force six or seven. On reaching the casualty, the skipper asked the lifeboat to stand by as he thought they could repair the engine. After an hour he asked the lifeboat to tow the vessel in. The trawler with her crew of five was taken in tow to Caherciveen. The lifeboat was back on station at 9.30 p.m.

Thirty-one Hours At Sea on Service

On a service beginning on 1 October 1971, the Valentia crew was at sea for thirty-one hours, standing by the Greek ship *George X*, broken down 65 miles south-west of the Mizen Lighthouse. The service was carried out in the relief lifeboat *Peter and Sarah Blake*, formerly stationed at Fenit, a boat of the 51 foot Barnett class, without a deck cabin or wheelhouse to protect the crew from the elements. A letter of commendation was sent to the station by the RNLI on this occasion.

Help for *Orion*

On 21 February 1972 the Irish Fishing Boat *Orion* sent a call for help. Her engine had failed 2½ miles east-south-east of Brandon Point. There was a north-easterly wind force three and a smooth sea. Visibility was 2 miles in mist. The lifeboat *Rowland Watts* slipped moorings at 11.15 p.m. After a four and a half hour passage she came up with the casualty, which had a crew of seven, 2 miles east-south-east of Brandon Point. At the skipper's request, the *Orion* was towed to her home port of Fenit. After some very welcome cups of tea from the skipper of the *Orion* the lifeboat returned to base and was again ready for service at 2 p.m.

Fouled Propeller

In an easterly wind and rough seas on 24 February 1972 the trawler *Ard Finbarr* got her propeller fouled by a trawl net. The *Rowland Watts* lifeboat slipped moorings at 7.25 a.m. in response to the distress call. There was fog, an easterly wind force five to six and reduced visibility. The casualty, with a crew of five, was found 5 miles south-west of Slea Head and was towed to Dingle at 12.30 p.m. The lifeboat was refueled and ready for service at 4.40 p.m.

Saved by a Flare

On 24 March 1972 in choppy seas and with overcast skies the lifeboat *Rowland Watts* slipped moorings at 7.35 p.m. This followed a report from Marcue at Cork

that a small boat was in distress near Ventry harbour. While searching the Ventry
Area a small hand flare was sighted approximately half a mile off the western
approach to Ventry. The lifeboat found the *Yorkshire Dory* with one man on board.
They landed the man and his craft at Ventry and returned to station. This was
the first service that a link call service was available via Valentia Radio. Honorary
Secretary Paddy Gallagher reported, 'Valentia Radio have now a link –call system
in operation and this with great assistance from Valentia Radio Staff is indeed a
great help'.

What Makes a Lifeboatman?

This is probably the question that most intrigues the landsman. In April 1972, Tony
Meade, a journalist with *The Kerryman* accompanied the *Rowland Watts* on one
mission and told his story under the title, 'A Night at Sea with the Valentia lifeboat':

> When the Honorary Secretary of Valentia Lifeboat, Paddy Gallagher, files his
> report to head office of the lifeboat service concerning the night of 5th/6th
> April 1972, it will probably read as follows: On the afternoon of 5th April a tel-
> ephone message was received from Haulbowline stating that a German Factory
> ship was heading for the South West Coast of Ireland with a very sick man on
> board. Valentia lifeboat was requested to rendezvous with the ship, Eric Weinert
> at 6.00 am on the morning of April 6th at 51 Degrees 30 minutes North and
> 10 Degrees 40 West. This was reached at about 5.00 am. At 6.10 am 'Rescue 53'
> reported to lifeboat that helicopter had taken sick man off. Lifeboat returned to
> base. No doubt Paddy Gallagher would never pen so inexact a report to his HQ,
> and equally, no doubt Cox. Dermot Walsh and his No. 2 Des Lavelle would not be
> so imprecise in their accounting for their twelve hours at sea. But for me, the situ-
> ation was somewhat different. This was my first experience of gale-force winds at
> sea; they varied from force three to eight and they treated the tiny 52' Rowland
> Watts with all the vigour they commanded. Lifeboats are not the most comfort-
> able of vessels. They are custom built to stand up to everything that the sea can
> throw at them, but they were not designed for human beings who must occupy
> them for many hours at a stretch. The entire fore part of the vessel is filled with
> two glistening diesel engines. Next comes the wheelhouse where strong men
> brace their legs against the movement of the sea. Aft, there is a small cabin with
> two bench type seats and adjustable chair for the radio–cum–radar man.
>   And behind this again comes a little oilskin covered cockpit opening directly
> into the cabin. I got to know this part of the boat quite well as it was here that
> my stomach endured its sea baptism. By midnight we were slipping down the
> harbour towards Portmagee Bridge. We had the benefit of the shelter provided
> by the harbour configuration, though, nevertheless, the crew went inside to

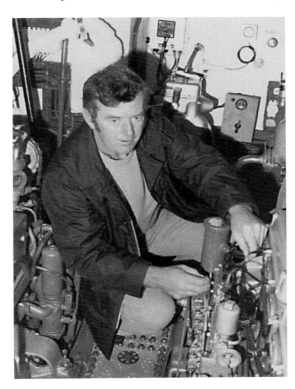

Joe Houlihan, mechanic, in the engine room of the *Rowland Watts*. Photo: courtesy of the RNLI.

avoid the heavy spray because at this point in time they had nothing better to do. I stayed on deck to see the bridge opening and to savour the spring of the boat once she met the rougher seas beyond. Never did a twenty five foot opening seem so small, a wave from the bridge operator and we headed to sea.

Surely, one of the greatest inventions is radar. While the coxswain handled the wheel Des Lavelle sat at his radar screen and called out changes of direction to him. One felt it was not necessary as Dermot Walsh must know the exit from Valentia Harbour like the proverbial back of his hand, but, nevertheless it was reassuring to see on screen the entire outline of the harbour and the bridge which we had so shortly left behind. Soon the Skelligs showed up ahead.

Risk for Many

Helmut Sranzen will never be more than a name to the men of Valentia Lifeboat. That he was in serious danger from peritonitis they did know, but they can not have known that he is just twenty-two years of age. They turned out to sea on the sort of night on which an ordinary chap is turning into his bed, grateful that he does not have to be out in the wind and misery of a wretched night. Others were occupied too. They were the men of Valentia Radio who would maintain contact with the lifeboat throughout the night, the men of the frigate *Banba* also racing to the scene. The RAF Shakleton Pilot. There was Rescue 53, who was in his bed when we were putting to sea, ready for a pre-dawn take off to the rendezvous position. There was the helicopter pilot of the Air Corps, also in bed when we struggled with the sea, wondering would the wind abate enough to enable him to lift off the German sailor in the morning. Aidan Walsh is just fifteen but is an experienced man of the sea. Son of the redoubtable Dermot, he went out with the lifeboat. A tall lad, he confessed readily that his stomach was not quite attuned to the conditions we met with. But only a landsman worries about being sick at sea; the experienced take it for granted, get it over with and get on with the job. And there was a bit of philosophy too, from the crewman who had a few pints earlier in the evening and now rued it. Guinness and a grumbling sea do not agree. By 4 a.m. the cold was beginning to bite through the oilskins and bulky anorak I wore underneath. A cup of something hot would have gone down well.

Dermot broke out some dry biscuits and a little bottle of rum. Those who could face it did. I wished I could, but could not. Two men slept on the floor of the cabin. Others of us lay on the benches, holding on with one hand to prevent the sea from having its way with us. At the feet of the helmsman two others lay on bench seats. All the time the diesels faultlessly throbbed, motor mechanic Joseph Houlihan checking the gauges, occasionally standing by the radio set as many calls came in from the German ship. There is an art to sleeping on a lifeboat. There is a way of wedging oneself in a corner so that the rolling and pitching of the boat does not dislodge one. The experts did it with ease. A combination of sheer discomfort and a determination to see all that was going on forced me awake most of the trip. By 5.15 a.m. we had reached the rendezvous position and the engines were cut back while the lifeboat waited.

Radio messages were frequently picked up, with the *Eric Weinert*, Rescue 53 and Valentia Radio talking back and forth. All the time a heavy swell was running, visibility from the low lying *Rowland Watts* was very limited.

Returned Home

The men of the lifeboat did not have the satisfaction of seeing the pick up of the sick man from the German ship. Indeed the *Eric Weinert* was not sighted at all. Rescue fifty-three reported to Valentia Radio that the pick up was complete and that the helicopter was on the way to the hospital. Then the Shakleton began to look for us, intending to take a photograph of the lifeboat. He gave up and headed home with a cheery goodbye. Des Lavelle replied, and notified Valentia Radio that we were going home. From the *Eric Weinert* a heavily accented voice thanked the lifeboat crew and wished us happy sailing. Twelve hours at sea and nothing noteworthy to report, except that the lifeboat was there when needed, ready to render any assistance it might be called upon to perform. And that is, I suppose, what the lifeboat service is all about. Back at Valentia the weary lifeboatmen began to carry five gallon jerry cans of oil the thirty yards to the moored *Rowland Watts*. Always first things first with the lifeboatmen. Then breakfast.

Dermot Walsh may have been slightly amused when I asked him what makes men put up with the gruelling demands of the service. He replied, like a man who had never asked himself the question, that it was a matter of great pride to have a lifeboat stationed there. There was a status in belonging to the crew. And then, thinking back on the night that had gone by, he said he could wish for a faster boat in view of the huge sea area Valentia Station covered, and with it, perhaps a little more comfort for the crew. Something that occurred to me as I watched the crew refuel the boat after the night's events was that a quay based tank for oil and a length of hose pipe would not go astray. After a twelve hour stint in heavy seas it would be very much appreciated.

Sick Lighthouse Keeper Landed

On 7 October 1972 the *Rowland Watts* was launched in choppy seas. This was in response to a request from Irish Lights to take a relief keeper to the Skelligs Rock Lighthouse and bring ashore a sick man. The lifeboat slipped moorings at 12.15 p.m. arrived at the rock at 2.10 p.m. and did the relief. She was back on station ready for service at 5.05 p.m.

Spanish Trawlers Assisted in Storm

When the Spanish trawlers *Monte Izankun* and *Costa de Isolda* sent out distress calls at 8.50 a.m. on the 9 November 1972 the *Rowland Watts* responded. The weather was appalling. There was a south-westerly storm force eight to ten. The sea was very rough and visibility was bad. Leaving the moorings at 9.15 a.m., the lifeboat encountered huge seas once she cleared Cromwell Point. Given the appalling conditions in the search area, Coxswain Walsh requested air assistance. An Aer Corps plane from Baldonnell and a RAF helicopter were tasked to assist. At 11 a.m. the trawlers were sighted and the aircraft were cancelled.

One trawler had all her fishing gear out to act as anchors. The other had complete engine failure. The lifeboat stood by. With two other Spanish trawlers coming to assist, the *Monte Izankun* informed the lifeboat that no further assistance was required in the area but requested that they stand by off the Cromwell's Point Lighthouse. Second Coxswain Des Lavelle spoke fluent Spanish so communications between the lifeboat and the casualty were made very easy as a result. The trawlers rudder was jammed. On arrival at Cromwell's Point, the lifeboat put a line to the trawlers starboard bow as she was veering to port. This was done at 4.30 p.m. and at 5.15 p.m. the lifeboat reported that the trawler was safe, with her fourteen crew, in Valentia harbour. The Honorary Secretary Mr Paddy Gallagher reported:

> I must add [to service report] that this indeed was an outstanding service by Coxswain Walsh and crew. They carried out a difficult task in terrible weather conditions. Again I must Compliment 2nd Coxswain Des Lavelle as he was a perfect interpreter with his fluent Spanish.

A letter of Commendation was sent to the station by the RNLI following this service.

Two Men Rescued from Beginish, Blaskets

On 2 February 1973 Marcue at Shannon reported sightings of a red flare and a fire on Beginish Island in the Blaskets Group of Islands. The *Rowland Watts* slipped moorings at 7.10 p.m., with the boarding boat in tow, and reached the search area at 8.45 p.m. Visibility was poor in drizzle. There was a westerly wind force four. Coxswain Walsh took the lifeboat close to the small island and fired a parachute flare. Two men were seen on the island. Second Coxswain Des Lavelle took charge of the boarding boat with three lifeboat men on board. The lifeboat kept the treacherous area lit with parachute flares as the boarding boat made her way to the island. Second Coxswain Lavelle kept the coxswain informed of progress by morse lamp.

One parachute flare was fired from the boarding boat as she negotiated a narrow inlet on the island. The two men, Gerard Fox from Co. Sligo and Steve Carwhile, were taken aboard the boarding boat and back to the lifeboat, which returned to base. Second Coxswain Des Lavelle remarked that a good big light flash lamp and a greater supply of parachute flares should be made available for this type of service.

Nurse from London Joins Crew

On 24 August 1973 a Greek cargo ship reported that she had a seriously injured crewman on board. She was approximately 5½ miles north-east of the Skelligs Rock. Coxswain Walsh was away from the island. At 9.30 a.m. the *Rowland Watts* slipped her moorings and put to sea with Second Coxswain Des Lavelle in charge. In a force five westerly wind and moderate seas the lifeboat reached the casualty.

A nurse, Miss Pauline Watts of Walcot Square, London, who was on an angling holiday, left the angling boat at Portmagee and joined the lifeboat. She very courageously went on board the ship and rendered assistance to the injured man.

The casualty was taken on board the lifeboat and was airlifted by the Air Corps from the lifeboat off Bray Head and taken to Tralee hospital. About two years earlier Miss Watts had been on an angling boat which the *Rowland Watts* had given assistance to, 'Miss Watts deserves the thanks of the crew and the RNLI,' remarked Honorary Secretary Paddy Gallagher.

Bereaved Lighthouse Keeper Landed

Two consecutive services by the *Rowland Watts* on 7 February 1974 and 12 April 1974 were to the Skelligs Rock Lighthouse. Both involved bringing lighthouse keeper Brian O'Regan ashore. On the first date his father had died and on the second date his mother had died. On the first date Coxswain Walsh reported big swells off the rock. Second Coxswain Des Lavelle volunteered to act as relief keeper at the lighthouse for a week. On the second occasion Coxswain Walsh was away and Second Coxswain Des Lavelle was in charge.

Don Muir towed to Portmagee

On 31 August 1974, the fishing vessel *Don Muir* experienced engine failure in St Finian's Bay. The lifeboat *City of Edinburgh*, on temporary duty at Valentia, slipped moorings at 8.25 a.m. Second Coxswain Des Lavelle was in charge. Motor Mechanic J.J. Houlihan attended for the service. Despite being on holiday, he was aware that the starboard engine had given trouble previously and went to sea. The trawler, with a crew of five, was reached at 9.50 a.m. The lifeboat having travelled via the opening span on Valentia Bridge. In a slight sea a towline was connected and the casualty and her crew landed at Portmagee pier.

Firemen and Pump Put Aboard Sinking Trawler

On 7 February 1975 the trawler *Spailpin Fanach* of Dublin, with six people on board, sent a distress call. She was taking water and in serious danger in a position 14 miles west-north-west of Bray Head. The lifeboat *John Gellatly Hyndman*, on temporary duty at Valentia, slipped moorings at 9.05 p.m. She embarked firemen and a portable motor pump at Renard pier and proceeded in rough seas to the casualty. The trawler *Patos Wish* was standing by the casualty. When the lifeboat arrived the casualty was very much down by the head, with the for'ard compartment flooded. Members of the Caherciveen fire brigade were life belted suitably and put on board with the pump. A Dingle trawler brought firemen from that town and a pump. As the water was pumped out *Patos Wish* took the casualty in tow and the lifeboat escorted her to Dingle. Coxswain Walsh remarked that the portable motor pump was mainly instrumental in saving the trawler. The crew also stated that the relief lifeboat was a beautiful boat and behaved absolutely perfectly.

Fishing Vessel Engine Failure

On 30 May 1975, Valentia Radio informed the honorary secretary that the fishing vessel *Rosebud*, with a crew of three, had experienced engine failure 10 miles north-west of Cromwell's Point Lighthouse on Valentia. The lifeboat *Rowland Watts* slipped moorings at 9.50 a.m. with Second Coxswain Des Lavelle in charge. In fine weather and a smooth sea the lifeboat reached the casualty at 11.10 a.m. and took her in tow to Caherciveen pier.

Three Services to the *Granat*

On 16 June 1975 the trawler *Granat*, skippered by Christy O'Shea of Valentia, had engine failure 10 miles north-north-west of the Wireless Point on Valentia. The *Rowland Watts* slipped her moorings at 4.30 p.m. in a force five westerly wind and a rough sea. At 6 p.m. the lifeboat took the casualty in tow. The lifeboat suffered some damage to the forehead bulwark on the port side. The casualty and her crew of five were landed at Valentia pier.

On 13 October 1975, the *Granat* had engine failure 6 miles north-north-west of Cromwell Point, Valentia . She was at the time returning to Valentia with an injured man. She had a crew of five. In very rough seas and a force seven south-easterly wind the *Rowland Watts* slipped her moorings at 1 p.m. with Second Coxswain Des Lavelle in Command. The trawler was taken in tow and landed at Valentia. The lifeboat was back at moorings ready for service at 5.30 p.m.

On 15 December 1975, misfortune befell the *Granat* again. While motoring to the fishing grounds she suffered engine failure near Cromwell Point Lighthouse. Her anchor was not holding. The distress call was received at 7.05 a.m., maroons were fired at 7.10 a.m. and the *Rowland Watts* slipped her moorings at 7.15 a.m. She reached the trawler with her five crew at 7.25 a.m. and took her in tow to Renard Point. Honorary Secretary P. Gallagher complimented Coxswain Dermot Walsh and the crew for their swift response to this distress call.

Help for *Ard Finbar*

On 9 March 1976, the fishing vessel *Ard Finbar* with a crew of four was in difficulties 1½ miles south of Lamb's Head in Kenmare Bay. Her steering was jammed.
In a rough sea and a southerly wind force seven to eight he called for immediate assistance. The lifeboat *Rowland Watts* slipped moorings at 8.30 a.m. and
proceeded via the Portmagee Channel. The honorary secretary had arranged for
Valentia Bridge to be opened and ready. The lifeboat reached the casualty at 11.15
a.m. The casualty was anchored at that time. She was taken in tow to Portmagee
pier.

Keeper Taken off Bull Rock in Difficult Conditions

On 8 May 1976, the Irish Lights Office requested the lifeboat evacuate a seriously ill light keeper from the Bull Rock Lighthouse. They assured the Honorary
Secretary Mr Gallagher that no helicopter was available to do the job. The *Rowland
Watts* under Coxswain Walsh put to sea at 6 p.m. with the large boarding boat in
tow. By arrangement, the Valentia Bridge was opened.
On arrival at the Bull Rock conditions were pretty rough, with a force four westerly wind. Second Coxswain Des Lavelle took charge of the boarding boat with
four lifeboatmen on board. After a number of attempts, he succeeded in getting
to the landing and taking the injured man, Brendan Copeland on board. They
returned to the lifeboat and the injured man was landed at Garnish and taken
to Bantry Hospital. In his comments on the service Honorary Secretary Mr P.
Gallagher wrote:

> Great credit is due to 2nd Cox. D. Lavelle for this service as darkness was setting
> in at the time and conditions at landing point on the Bull Rock were pretty
> treacherous. Sick man on derrick end actually dipped in the swell [sea] on two
> occasions before being finally got into the boarding boat.

Lifeboat Away in Five Minutes

On 10 May 1976 the trawler *Johnny Ruth*, with a crew of four on board, suffered
engine failure. With a moderate sea and a north-north-westerly wind force six
she was very close to the shore at Beginish at the entrance to Valentia harbour.
The alarm was raised at 12.50 p.m. Coxswain Dermot Walsh, Second Coxswain
Des Lavelle and Mechanic Joseph Houlihan were all on the pier. Des Lavelle
used his motor boat to ferry the crew to the lifeboat. The lifeboat *Rowland Watts*
slipped moorings at 12.55 p.m and went to the assistance of the trawler which

was anchored quite close to the rocks. She was taken in tow to Renard pier. Mr Gallagher remarked, 'This service was I am sure the quickest ever carried out and the crew who were in close proximity to the pier launched 938 in record time'.

Nurse Put on Board Trawler

On 11 December 1976 the lifeboat *Rowland Watts* put to sea with Nurse Daly of Valentia Hospital on board. They were responding to a call from the trawler *Spailpin Fanach*, which had a seriously injured man on board. While *en route* they received a message from the trawler *Pato's Wish* that there was a man overboard from the trawler *St Colette* near Black head. Nurse Daly was put on aboard the *Spailpin Fanach* and the lifeboat went to the new search area. Despite the efforts of the lifeboat, eight other vessels, a helicopter and a plane, the man, unfortunately, was not found.

Trawler Towed Home

On 23 June 1977, following a distress call from the trawler *Granat*, the *Rowland Watts* lifeboat was launched. In good weather and a slight sea the lifeboat, under Second Coxswain Des Lavelle slipped moorings at 10.05 a.m. The casualty was reached at 11.35 a.m., 11½ miles west of Cromwell's Point. A tow line was connected and the vessel was towed to Valentia harbour.

Lifeboat Takes Over Tow from *Béal Bocht*

On 20 September 1977 Valentia Radio informed the honorary secretary that the fishing boat *Béal Inse* was dragging its anchor quite close to shore at Reenadroulaun Point. With Joseph Houlihan in charge, the lifeboat *Rowland Watts* slipped moorings at 5.45 p.m. in a rough sea and force four northerly wind. At 6.15 p.m. the lifeboat reached the casualty, which was in tow of Des Lavelle's fishing vessel *Béal Bocht*. The tow was transferred to the lifeboat and the casualty was towed to Valentia. The fishing vessel *Pluto* also gave help to the casualty.

Ships Lifeboat Recovered

Early on the morning of the 14 October 1977, following a report that a ship's lifeboat with ten people on board was drifting helplessly off Ballydavid Head, the *Rowland Watts'* lifeboat slipped her moorings. In a south-westerly wind, force five and a moderate sea, the lifeboat proceeded to the casualty area. When the lifeboat reached the position 1½ miles north of Dún Na Capple they found the casualty upside down. They recovered it and returned it to the tug *Afon Goch*. The master of the tug told Coxswain Dermot Walsh that he had been towing the cargo ship *Skyhope*. A row developed between the crews. One man, who had been seriously injured, was being conveyed ashore in the ship's lifeboat, the boat capsized and the crew was rescued by a local fishing boat. The injured man had since died. Following this service the manager, F.P. Mawdsely of Holyhead Towing Co. Ltd, Newry Beach Yard Holyhead sent £50 to the Valentia Branch Funds and £50 to the crew.

Workmen on Inisvickalane Given Provisions and Lifeboat Crew's Spirits Raised

On 8 December 1977, the light keepers on Inistearaght lighthouse reported seeing distress flares on Inisvickalane. It was known that workmen were working on a house there for then Minister for Health Mr Charles J. Haughey. The *Rowland Watts*, under Coxswain Dermot Walsh, set out at 9 p.m. with the boarding boat in tow. On arriving at the island, parachute flares were fired and the boarding boat party safely made their way in treacherous conditions to the beach. The workmen told them they had lost radio contact with the mainland. They had very little food. The lifeboat crew gave them supplies and made arrangements for them to be taken off the island the following morning by helicopter. On hearing of the service, Mr Haughey rewarded the crew with twelve bottles of rum.

In 1978 there were eight launches. Only one effective service was on 12 July 1978. An ill man was landed from a Spanish trawler.

Rosebud Towed to Safety

On 20 June 1979 the fishing vessel *Rosebud*, with a crew of three, was fishing for lobsters near Inishnabro, in the Blaskets group of islands. Her propeller became fouled by a rope and she was disabled. The *Rowland Watts* lifeboat slipped her moorings in fine weather. She found the casualty 1½ miles north-west of Inishnabro. A tow line was put on board and she was towed to Caherciveen pier.

Fishing Boat with Four People Towed in

On 10 July 1979, the Gardaí at Caherciveen reported to the honorary secretary that a vessel appeared to be in difficulties in Kells Area. Mr Gallagher, the honorary secretary, checked with T. O'Sullivan of Kells who had made the report to the Gardaí. The *Rowland Watts* slipped her moorings at 9.50 p.m. and made for the casualty area. At 11.30 p.m. the lifeboat found the fishing vessel *Jacqdaw* of Dublin with four people on board drifting in a choppy sea and a force four south-south-westerly wind. She was 1½ miles north of Foileye Point. A tow line was passed across and she was towed into Kells Bay.

Béal Inse Towed to Safety

Six days later, on 16 July, a distress call was received by Valentia Radio from the fishing vessel *Béal Inse* that she had engine failure in the Blaskets Sound. She needed immediate assistance. The *Rowland Watts* lifeboat slipped moorings with Second Coxswain/Mechanic Joseph Houlihan in charge at 12.20 p.m. In poor visibility and a choppy sea the casualty was located at 2.10 p.m. A towline was passed across and the vessel, which had a crew of four, was towed to safety at Valentia.

Position Unsure

On 7 September 1979, in a rough sea and nil visibility the fishing vessel *Orion* of Dublin failed to identify Doulous Head and was unsure of its position. The *Rowland Watts* lifeboat slipped moorings at 9 p.m. and set course for the area north-west of Valentia Lighthouse. Coxswain Dermot Walsh contacted the casualty and requested him to fire a parachute flare and the lifeboat also fired one. The casualty reported the lifeboat flare south of him. The lifeboat picked up the casualty on radar ¾ mile away. She escorted the casualty into Valentia harbour.

Survivors Landed at Ventry

Two days later, on 9 September 1979, the *Rowland Watts* was at sea again. The Gardaí at Dingle reported that the 21 foot fishing vessel *Lady Jane* had hit rocks on the east side of Inishnabro in the Blaskets. At 8 p.m. the casualty informed Second Coxswain/Mechanic Joseph Houlihan that his vessel had sunk and both occupants were marooned on the island. The lifeboat had the boarding boat in tow. Three of the crew went ashore and brought the two survivors to the lifeboat. They were landed at Ventry pier.

Yacht Saved

On 4 April 1980 the motor yacht *Nachrista* was reported by Valentia Radio, to have engine failure 4 miles north of Cromwell's Point Lighthouse. The crew were working on boats in the vicinity of the station. The lifeboat *Rowland Watts* launched 11.20 a.m. with Second Coxswain/Mechanic Joseph Houlihan in charge. The casualty was reached at 12 p.m. and towed at reduced speed to Valentia pier. Mrs Krisac, wife of the owner of the casualty, gave a gift of £20 to the crew.

Minister for Justice Reported Vessel in Distress

Justice Minister Gerard Collins was sent a letter from the RNLI thanking him for alerting the lifeboat to the plight of a fishing boat in difficulty on 4 May 1980. The director wrote on 15 December 1980:

> Dear Mr Collins.
> Following the recent receipt of the report concerning the service carried out by the Valentia Lifeboat to the motor fishing vessel 'Welcome Home' on the 4th May 1980, I write to express to you The Institution's warm and appreciative thanks for first reporting the plight of the motor fishing vessel to our Honorary Secretary at Valentia and then keeping him informed of the position of the casualty at regular intervals. The help was much appreciated by all concerned with the lifeboat station and I wish to add my personal thanks.
> Yours sincerely,
> W. J. Graham,
> Director.

The casualty, with a crew of three, was found drifting towards Rossbeigh Strand by the *Rowland Watts* in very rough seas. A towline was connected with some difficulty and the casualty was towed to Coonana harbour.

Lifeboat Stands by Vessel in Storm

On the 18 December 1980 the tanker *Authenticity* of London with a crew of eight suffered engine failure. Her anchors were not holding and in north-westerly wind force ten to eleven she was in grave danger of being driven ashore. She was 4 miles north-west of Smerwick. After assembling at 1.15 a.m. the crew found it impossible to get on board the lifeboat. Donal Walsh, a local fisherman, took the crew in his fishing boat and put them on board the lifeboat *Rowland Watts*. Seas were breaking across the *Sheithe Line* – all across the mouth of Valentia harbour

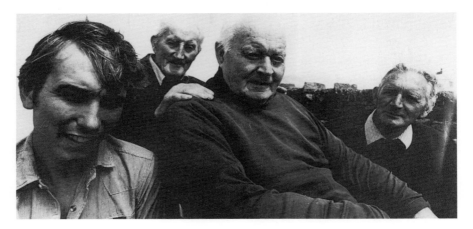

Four coxswains, Seanie Murphy, Jack Sugrue, Jeremiah O'Connell and Dermot Walsh. Photo: Courtesy of the *Sunday Press*.

between Cromwell's Point and Beginish Island. Half speed had to be maintained all the way to the casualty in the atrocious conditions. The lifeboat was with the casualty at 5 a.m. and stood by until 12.50 p.m. At that time the Captain of the Casualty reported that the engines were satisfactorily repaired and that no further assistance was required. The lifeboat was ready for service again at 4.30 p.m., after 14.75 gruelling hours.

Fishing Vessel Picked up Distress Signal

On 13 June 1981 the fishing vessel MFV *Béal Inse*, berthed at Valentia pier picked up a VHF distress message. The Fishing Vessel *Interceptor* had engine failure and was afraid dragging her anchor in the Blaskets (Inishvickallane) Sound. In rough sea and west-southerly wind force seven the relief lifeboat *Euphrosyne Kendal* set out with Coxswain Dermot Walsh in command. In rough seas, strong tide and poor visibility the casualty with a crew of three was located. A line was put on board and she was towed to Valentia pier. At that time, Valentia Radio did not have VHF so it was fortunate that the message was picked up by the *Béal Inse*.

Dermot Walsh retired from the position of coxswain at the end of 1981. During his tenure of office, Valentia lifeboat launched a total of 111 times and saved seventy lives. 'The new lifeboat due for Valentia in 1983 will be looking for a young crew. It was nice to be involved,' Dermot told *The Kerryman* newspaper. 'I'll be there in spirit all the time. It is all voluntary and you feel you are helping your own kind at sea'. Seanie Murphy succeeded Dermot Walsh as coxswain in 1982, Seanie, then twenty-six, was unusual in RNLI terms in that his first position on the lifeboat was that of coxswain.

Hurricane Service Welcomes New Coxswain

A force eleven south-wester was his introduction. On the night of 11 March 1982 the 1,400 ton refitted Spanish ship MV *Ranga* was on her maiden voyage from Valencia in Spain to Iceland. Due to engine failure, the *Ranga* was swept on to the rocks at treacherous Coomenole on the western end of the Dingle Peninsula. The *Rowland Watts* launched at 10.45 p.m. and arriving off the casualty assisted the Dingle Coast Lifesaving unit and an RAF helicopter by illuminating the area with parachute flares. Seven men were pulled ashore by the Coast Lifesaving Service. The RAF helicopter airlifted the other eight men to safety. The Minister for Transport wrote the following letter of commendation to the Irish District Office of the RNLI:

> Lt. Col. Brian Clark,
> Royal National Lifeboat Institution,
> 10 Merrion Square,
> Dublin 2.
>
> Dear Lt. Col. Clark,
> On the night of the 11/12 March last the Spanish Vessel 'Ranga' went aground at Coomeenole Bay off the Dingle Peninsula. Notwithstanding the very difficult conditions at the time the entire crew of the grounded vessel were brought to safety. The Valentia Lifeboat was launched and was present at the scene of the casualty. While the physical conditions were such that the lifeboat was not able to intervene directly, it stood by, firing illuminating flares for a RAF. helicopter as it approached the shipwreck, while rescue operations were successfully effected by the Coast Lifesaving Service and the RAF helicopter. The fact that the shipwreck did not involve any loss of life was due to the combined efforts of the various agencies involved. I would be grateful if you would convey to the crew of the Valentia Lifeboat and all those connected with it, my thanks and appreciation of their vital contribution to the rescue operations.
> Yours sincerely,
> John Wilson,
> Minister for Transport.

The *Rowland Watts* launched on ten further services after the *Ranga* from Valentia before being transferred to the reserve fleet. Her final lifesaving service was on 22 August 1982 when she saved the fishing vessel *Shooting Star* of Tralee and her two occupants. In all, the *Rowland Watts* had launched on service from Valentia 158 times and had saved 132 people.

Rowland Watts, the donor of the legacy which funded this lifeboat, lived at Colchester in Essex, England. It is probable that he never set foot in Valentia and possible that he never even heard of it, but through his generosity 132 people were saved from certain death on the Kerry Coast and his name will be remembered through his generous gift for a long time to come. There is no finer epitaph: 'This Man Gave Life to Others'. The departure of this lifeboat also marked the end of another era. The traditional wooden-hulled lifeboats of this type were the culmination of 150 years' experience of wooden boat building, design and craftsmanship. Research begun in the 1960s had led to the introduction in the 1970s, of fast, more manoeuvrable, more comfortable self-righting lifeboats made of steel, glass-reinforced plastic and aluminium.

The *Rowland Watts* is now back at Valentia. A fund has been created with a view to restoring her. She was the first motor lifeboat built specifically for Valentia.

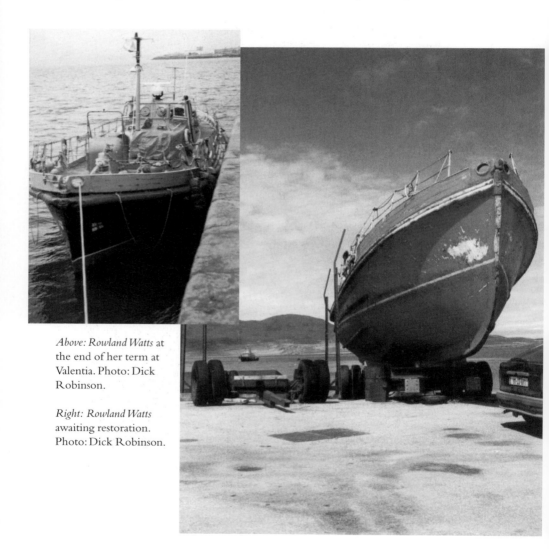

Above: Rowland Watts at the end of her term at Valentia. Photo: Dick Robinson.

Right: Rowland Watts awaiting restoration. Photo: Dick Robinson.

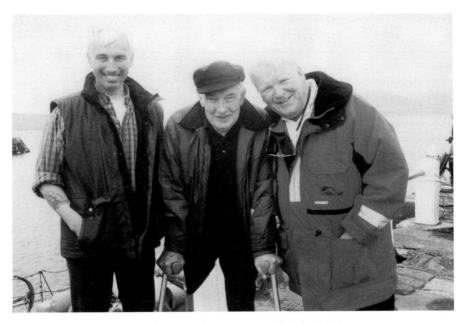

Seanie, his dad, Sean and Derek Davis. Photo: courtesy of Adrian Mackey.

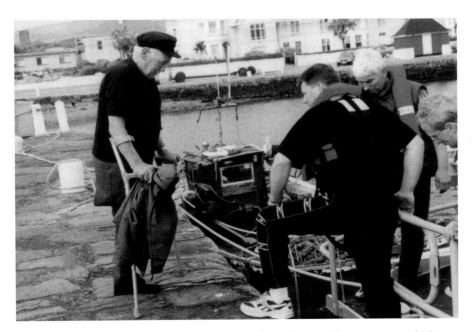

Sean Murphy, Leo Houlihan, Seanie Murphy and Johnny Quigley. Photo: courtesy of Adrian Mackey.

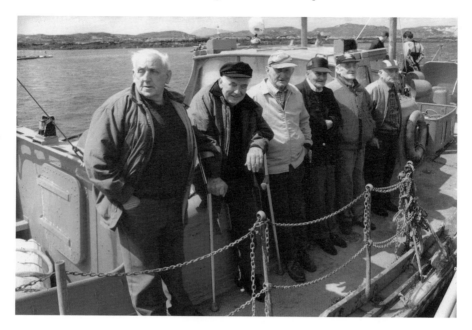

John Shanahan, Sean Murphy, Dodie Walsh, Miko Leary, Tony Walsh and Eddie Murphy. Photo: courtesy of Adrian Mackey.

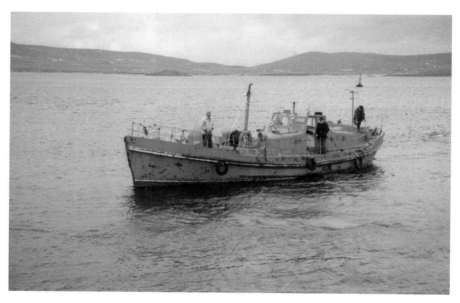

Rowland Watts' last voyage on 28 May 1999. Photo: courtesy of Adrian Mackey.

EIGHT

A NEW ARUN CLASS LIFEBOAT – *MARGARET FRANCES LOVE*

On the 18 February 1983 at 4 p.m. the *Rowland Watts* lay hove to off Cromwells Point Lighthouse. The new lifeboat, *Margaret Frances Love*, swept down close to her port side, and a ragged cheer broke out on board the old lifeboat. There was many a tear of joy, and pride, and nostalgia, as other times and other men were recalled. But the over-riding emotion was pride in the Valentia Lifeboat Station and in this new vessel which would increase its lifesaving potential. While it will never be totally safe, lifeboating in the area would be less dangerous. The differences between the two boats were stark. The traditionally built *Rowland Watts* lay low in the water while the new boat planed over it at double the speed. The *Rowland Watts* escorted the new lifeboat home. Her passage crew was Seanie Murphy, coxswain; Richard Connolly, second coxswain; Jimmy Murphy; Martin Moriarty; and Padraig Ring. The district inspector, Mr T. Course, and district engineer were also on board. They had been diverted while on passage to a casualty, the *Billet* with a crew of three. The vessel had machinery failure one mile west of Mizen Head. The lifeboat was 5 miles north-west of Dursey Sound and altered course immediately. On arriving at the casualty area the fishing vessel *Marden* was alongside the casualty. She took the *Billet* in tow to Castletownbere and the lifeboat resumed her passage to Valentia.

French Trawler Assisted

The *Margaret Frances Love* launched on her first service at Valentia on 9 April 1983 when she assisted the fishing boat *Kalernec* of France. The vessel, which had a fouled propeller, was landed at Valentia. Former Second Coxswain Des Lavelle sailed with the lifeboat as he is a fluent French speaker.

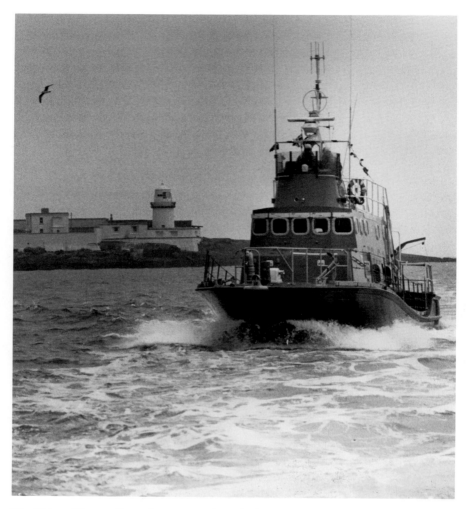

The lifeboat *Margaret Frances Love* enters Valentia harbour for the first time, leaving Cromwell's Point lighthouse to starboard, 18 February 1983. Photo: courtesy of the *Cork Examiner*.

The Naming Ceremony: 17 September 1983

The morning sunshine gave hope that the blustery weather of the previous few days had cleared up. Fishermen and lifeboat men prophesied rain for the afternoon, and sure enough, shortly before the naming ceremony began the wind picked up and the rain began. The hundreds of guests and islanders huddled in the shelter of the pier's short wall. At precisely 2 p.m. the platform party began to arrive. Lady Killanin, who was to name the boat, was presented with flowers by Rosemary Quigley, daughter of the deputy launching authority. Having been introduced to the youthful crew of the lifeboat, the party moved on to the platform and the proceedings were opened by Father Denis Costelloe, the Branch Chairman. Thanking all the guests for coming from far and wide, Fr Costelloe bade a particular welcome to Lt Commander Brian Miles, then deputy Director of the RNLI. The lifeboat was handed into the care of the station by Mr Clayton Love, a Vice President of RNLI Mr P.J. Gallagher, Station Honorary Secretary, accepted the boat and noted with some sadness the passing of the *Rowland Watts*.

Most Revd Dr Kevin McNamara, Bishop of Kerry; and Revd Brian Lougheed, Rector of Killarney; blessed the lifeboat. Lady Killanin named the lifeboat, *Margaret Frances Love* and the choir sang 'Sing to the Mountains, Sing to the Sea'. Coxswain Seanie Murphy invited the platform party for a cruise in the lifeboat and they were joined by Dermot Walsh, who had been presented with a framed certificate marking his retirement after thirty-two years service with the Valentia lifeboat. Former Coxswains Jeremiah O'Connell and Jack Sugrue attended the ceremony as did representatives of ten other lifeboat stations. With the weather at its worst, and torrential rain in continuous downpour, the excellent salmon buffet laid on by the ladies of the island in the former Western Union Office building was both refreshing and welcome.

Dancing Wave Saved

On 28 September 1983 the fishing vessel *Dancing Wave* of Cork sprung a leak near the North Landing on Inistearaght. She had a crew of three and needed urgent assistance. The lifeboat *Margaret Frances Love* with Second Coxswain Richard Connolly

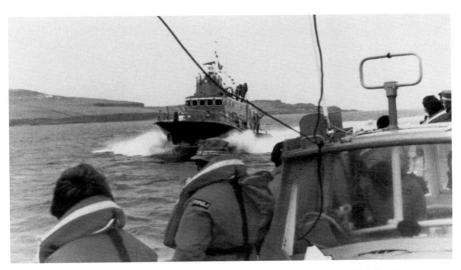

The *Rowland Watts* meeting the *Margaret Frances Love* off Valentia. Photo: Dick Robinson, on 18 February 1983.

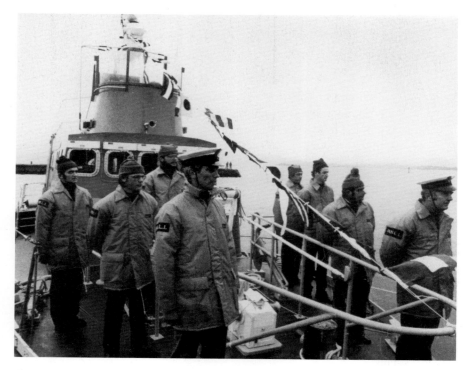

Coxswain Sean Murphy, Mechanic Joseph Houlihan and crew during the naming ceremony, 17 September 1983. Photo: courtesy of the *Kerryman*.

in charge slipped her moorings at 3.12 p.m. There was a moderate choppy sea, fog and poor visibility. The fishing vessels, *Béal Bocht* and *Ros Conlon* also went to the assistance of the casualty. On arrival at the scene the coxswain decided to use the emergency portable pump to stem the flow of water. This was very effective. The lifeboat crew and others at the scene managed to curb the leak (from the stern tube) sufficiently to enable the casualty to be towed to Portmagee pier.

First Lifesaving Service

On 3 May 1984, what was deemed to be the first lifesaving service by the new lifeboat took place. In a south-easterly force six to eight wind, rough seas and a 15 foot swell the *Marita Ann* sent out a distress call. She was 12 miles west of Loop Head and 18 miles north of Brandon. She had a crew of three and nets had fouled her propeller. Slipping Moorings at 4.30 p.m. *Margaret Frances Love* was abeam of the casualty at 7.30 p.m. The wind was now a full force eight with a corresponding sea. Coxswain Murphy decided not to go alongside the casualty but received a tow line from her. Using a steel hawser from the casualty and securing it and the

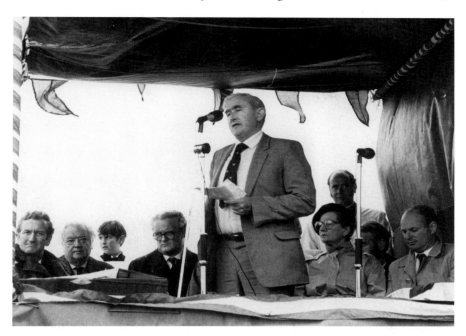

Above: Paddy
Gallagher, station
honorary secretary
since 1968 addressing
the assembled guests
and spectators at the
naming ceremony.
Photo: courtesy of the
Kerryman.

Right: Lord Killanin
makes presentation to
ex Coxswain Dermot
Walsh. Paddy Gallagher
in centre.

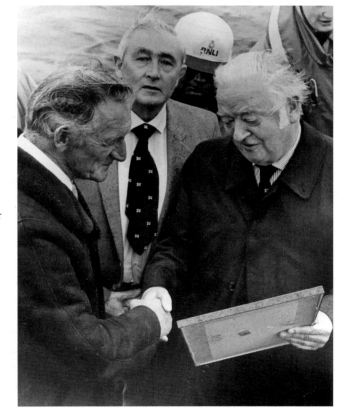

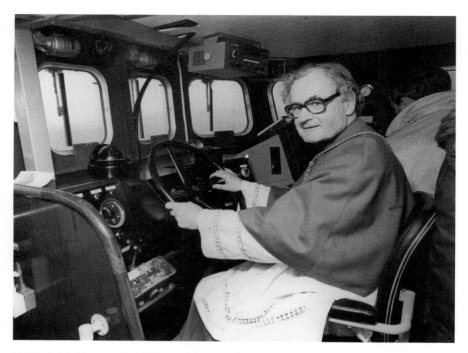

Dr Kevin McNamara, then Bishop of Kerry, on board the *Margaret Frances Love* on 17 September 1983. Photo: courtesy of the *Kerryman*.

lifeboats tow rope to a heavy tyre, ensuring flexibility in the tow, the casualty was towed to Fenit where she was put safely alongside at 1 a.m. The lifeboat was back at moorings and ready for service 5 a.m.

Fifty-Five Mile Passage to Casualty

On 14 July 1984, Valentia Radio received a distress call from the Motor Fishing Vessel *Ardent II* of Castletownbere. She was west of Loop Head with a fouled propeller. She had a crew of six. Fifteen minutes after the alarm was raised the lifeboat Margaret Frances Love slipped moorings at 1.15 p.m. In a north-westerly wind force four to six and a rough sea she set out on the fifty-five mile journey.

Arriving at the position 52.45 north 10.50 west at 4.35 p.m. a towline was connected to the casualty. Coxswain Seanie Murphy decided to tow the forty-ton vessel to Fenit which was the nearest safe port. The tow was slow, at just six knots. The tow parted after fifty minutes but was reconnected. The vessel and her six crew were safely landed at Fenit at 1 a.m. The lifeboat refuelled and returned to Valentia. She was back at moorings at 8.15 a.m. on the 15 July, after over nineteen hours at sea and six lives saved.

A Close-Run Thing

On 17 September 1984, the rescue of the *Interceptor* with a crew of three was a close-run thing. The fishing vessel had a fouled propeller and was very near Doulous Head. Thirteen minutes after launching in a rough sea and north-westerly wind force four to six, the *Margaret Frances Love* reached the casualty. A tow line was quickly passed across and the casualty was towed safely into Valentia harbour.

Letter of Thanks from Chief of Operations

The fishing vessel *Fortune Hunter*, due in Ventry at 4 p.m. on the 12 January 1985, had not arrived by 7.30 p.m. The Gardaí notified the honorary secretary at Valentia. At 7.50 p.m. the *Margaret Frances Love* slipped her moorings under the command of Coxswain Seanie Murphy. The wind was south-easterly force six. The casualty had left Cromane at 1.30 p.m. and therefore the coxswain decided to search the Ventry area first and then work eastwards back along the rugged and dangerous Dingle Peninsula. The *Fortune Hunter* was located in shallow water very close to Bull Head. A line was passed and the vessel was taken in tow to Dingle. A letter from the Chief of Operations was sent to thank the coxswain and crew for their efficiency during the service. If the *Rowland Watts* had sailed into a disaster in her early days with the *Marie Brigette*, the disaster which carried the *Margaret Frances Love* 112 miles from station was to be one of indescribable horror.

Air India Disaster: A Harrowing Service

The speck that represented Air India flight 182 disappeared from the screen at Shannon Air Traffic Control at 8.13 a.m. on 26 June 1985. The news reached Valentia, Baltimore, Courtmacsherry and Ballycotton by the explosive summons of maroons, so often the harbinger of disaster. All four lifeboats launched, the latter three being recalled. A boarding party from the Irish Naval vessel L.E. *Aisling* inspecting the catch on board a Spanish trawler saw their ship pick up way and sail westwards without them. Coxswain Seanie Murphy, Second Coxswain Richard Connolly, Mechanic Joseph Houlihan, Assistant Mechanic James Murphy and Seamus and Eamon Murphy with Shane O'Neill and Nealie Lyne reached the blood-red shark-infested search area. They were to recover five bodies, one that of a five-year-old child. Those who were parents amongst the lifeboat crew wept openly and unashamedly. A child is everybody's child. Through good navigation and conservation of fuel the lifeboat got to the then manned Skelligs Rock, where the lighthouse keepers gave enough fuel to complete the journey to Valentia.

In the sombre Monday dawn light the lifeboat crept into Knightstown pier Sergeant Patrick Reidy, Dr Alan O'Sullivan, Nurse Joan Daly and three soldiers were embarked. Despite the exhaustion and trauma, Coxswain Murphy moved the lifeboat away from the pier to allow the medical examination to take place and to have the bodies prepared for transport to Cork by the Army and Gardaí.

A simple enough gesture in itself, seeing to it that these tragic people torn from life, half a world from home by a bomb placed by some mindless maniac, were treated in death with as much dignity as the circumstances allowed, was a credit to the coxswain, his crew and the RNLI as a whole. For their part in this service, a letter of commendation was sent to the station by the Chief of Operations.

Taurima sinks at Mizen Head

On 7 October 1985 the *Margaret Frances Love* launched to the assistance of the yacht *Taurima*. This had struck rocks at Mizen Head. Aboard was Mr Charles J. Haughey and four other people. When Valentia lifeboat was 12 miles from the casualty word was received that all the people were safe aboard the Baltimore lifeboat. Valentia lifeboat returned to station.

Lifeboat and Land Based Rescue Services Save Delores O'Connor

The 9 November 1985, was to see the lifeboat back at the Dingle Peninsula again in an incident which brought together every rescue agency in the vicinity of Annascaul: the lifeboat, Tralee Fire Brigade, Kerry Mountain Rescue Team, the Gardaí, a plant hire contractor and a courageous group of local citizens. Frightening in the simplicity of its happening, highly dramatic for its duration and happy in its outcome, it is the story of Delores O'Connor. She had joined her father in the familiar routine of rounding up the sheep. While seventeen-year-old Delores was crossing some huge clifftop rocks which had been dumped during earlier road works, the rocks suddenly shifted, slipped and at the end of a miniature landslide the girl was trapped beneath great slabs. The only way to release Delores was to lift one huge rock vertically above her and the only subsequent way out was down the cliff to Bananeer Strand.

When air blankets from the Tralee Fire Brigade had lifted some of the rocks, a scaffold had to be erected, a net was slung from the scaffold and placed around the endangering rock. Trapped since 4 p.m., she was not taken clear until 9.40 p.m. She was carried to the lifeboat dinghy which was waiting at the bottom of the cliff and her stretcher was carefully placed aboard and she was ferried up the coast to a suitable landing place. There she was handed into the care of an ambulance crew and taken to Tralee General Hospital, where she made a complete recovery.

Patrick Sarsfield Towed to Safe Anchorage

On 27 May 1986 the weather was extremely bad. There was a west–north–westerly wind, force nine, very high seas and generally poor conditions. The sailing yacht *Patrick Sarsfield*, with a crew of five was dragging her anchor at Smerwick and the owner was fearful for the safety of the vessel and her crew.

The lifeboat *Margaret Frances Love* slipped moorings at 8.30 a.m. Despite very heavy seas in the Blaskets Sound area the lifeboat came up with the casualty at 10.10 a.m. She was towed to a safe anchorage at Smerwick. The owner of the yacht, Mr Gerry Locke, who is a shoreline member was pleased with the assistance given. He made a gift of £50 to the branch funds and a gift of £30 to the crew. Both Coxswain Murphy and the crew were delighted with the way the lifeboat behaved in extreme conditions.

Countessa Viv Sinks

'Countessa Viv Sinks', 'Lifeboat Leads Search After Trawler Sinks' 'Hopes Fade for Five Fishermen'; these were the headlines in the *Evening Echo* on 2 August 1986. The *Countessa Viv* sank in a mysterious accident at Fair Head at the entrance to Castletownbere harbour. On the evening of the 1 August 1986 Valentia lifeboat slipped moorings at 6.30 p.m. She set out in south–south–westerly winds force seven to nine. The sea was rough and visibility was poor. On reaching the casualty area at 9.05 p.m the lifeboat encountered very high seas and twenty to 25 foot swells. The Lowestoft registered *Countessa Viv* was Spanish owned. She had a crew of fifteen. She was long lining for hake and made for Castletownbere when the storm broke. She sank in twenty-six meters of water after striking the rocks. Ten of the crew were rescued by local boats. The search for the other five led by the lifeboat was continued until darkness and again at first light the following morning, Irish and British helicopters and local boats all assisted but the five were not found and presumed drowned. The lifeboat returned to moorings some twenty-four hours after setting out having endured some of the worst conditions that the Atlantic could throw at her.

American Yacht Towed in Bad Weather

The yacht American *Signet*, with two on board, was unsure of her position on 25 August 1986. Following a link call via Valentia Radio he was given his position by the coxswain and a course for Bray Head. He stated that he needed no further assistance. Forty minutes later at 12.30 p.m. the skipper asked for assistance. The *Margaret Frances Love* set out in bad weather, force eight to ten north-westerly wind, very rough seas and fifteen to 20 foot swells. The casualty was 14 miles from station, north-west of the Skelligs. With some difficulty in the conditions a tow line was connected and the yacht and her two crew were towed to Portmagee and safety.

Launch in Phenomenal Seas

When the Italian tanker *Capo Emma* got into difficulty at 51.54 north 12.04 west on 18 November 1986 the *Margaret Frances Love* was launched. The wind was force eight to ten north-westerly. Seas were described as phenomenal. The swells were 30 to 40 feet. The casualty gained the shelter of Bantry Bay and the lifeboat was recalled.

Casualty with Ill Crew Escorted to Safe Harbour

Less than a month later, on 16 December 1986, a distress call was received from the Spanish Trawler *Faro Sillero*. She was in a position 51.56 north 10.38 west. The weather was bad with very high seas and 20 to 25 foot swells. The sea was breaking across the entrance to the harbour at Cromwell's Point. With great skill and caution, Coxswain Seanie Murphy brought the *Margaret Frances Love* out to the open sea. On arriving at the casualty it was agreed that to attempt a transfer in such conditions would be extremely hazardous. The lifeboat, streaming the drogue, escorted the casualty into harbour. Here, in the more sheltered water, the two men were taken on board the lifeboat and landed at Renard pier where they were handed into the care of the waiting ambulance crew and taken to Tralee Hospital. The first of the nineteen launches of Valentia lifeboat for the year 1987 – a selection of which will be recalled – was on 14 March 1987.

Vessel Located in Dense Fog

The small vessel *Kilkee Lass* with a crew of three was on passage from Castletownbere to Kilkee. In fair weather and slight sea but dense fog she was unsure of her position. At 10 a.m. the *Margaret Frances Love* slipped her moorings. Coxswain Murphy contacted the casualty by radio and using the radar reached her at 10.20 a.m. She was in dangerous ground, near Culloo on the north side of Valentia. The lifeboat escorted the casualty to the safety of Valentia harbour.

The skipper was totally inexperienced and was using a road map for navigation purposes.

Doctor Taken Out to Ship

On 5 May the trawler *San Paulo*, which was 3 miles west of the Skelligs, requested medical assistance for a seriously injured crewman. Slipping moorings at 11.45 a.m. the lifeboat *Margaret Frances Love* embarked Dr Alan O'Sullivan at Renard pier and set out for the casualty. On reaching the casualty at 12.45 p.m. the injured man was transferred to the lifeboat. He was treated by Dr O'Sullivan and landed at Renard pier where he was transferred to a waiting ambulance and taken to Tralee Regional Hospital.

Historic Lifeboat of 'Daunt Rock Rescue Fame' Towed in

On 19 July 1987 a former Limerick Harbour Commissioners pilot boat with a crew of three was in difficulties 4½ miles north-west of Black Head Sound. She was in fact the former lifeboat *Mary Stanford* (ON 733) which had been purchased for preservation by Brendan Sliney, grandson of Patsy Sliney who carried out the Daunt Rock service in this vessel. The lifeboat (relief) *Margaret Russell Frazer* slipped moorings at 11.08 a.m. and set out for the casualty in rough seas in north-north-westerly wind force five to seven. Very rough seas were encountered in the Blaskets Sound. The casualty was reached at 2.20 p.m. and towed to Valentia. Former Coxswain Dermot Walsh (Silver Medalist) accompanied the crew on this trip and was very impressed with the performance of the Arun class boat.

Towline connected in Heavy Seas

On 12 December 1987 the *Ronan Padraig* of Tralee with a crew of six had a fouled propeller 42 miles west of the Blaskets. After setting out for the casualty, the lifeboat *Margaret Frances Love* encountered an oil leak between the gearbox and the cooler. She returned to Valentia where mechanic Joseph Houlihan made up a new pipe and repaired the leak. At 3.55 p.m. the lifeboat set out again. She reached the casualty at 7.15 p.m. In easterly wind force six to eight and rough seas with 10 to 15 foot swells a tow line was connected. The vessel was towed, in a slow tow, to Valentia arriving at 8.55 a.m.

In 1988 the lifeboat launched nine times.

Saved in Blaskets Sound

Five lives were saved on the 23 July 1988. The sailing yacht *Turnabout* with five on board was drifting towards rocks at Clogher Head, in the Blaskets Sound. Her anchor was not holding. In rough sea and poor visibility the lifeboat *Margaret Frances Love* slipped moorings at 4.22 p.m. With Second Coxswain Richard Connolly in charge she reached the casualty an hour later. She was taken in tow to Valentia pier.

Triumph and Tragedy on Friday the Thirteenth

Friday 13 January 1989 opened on the Kerry coast with a most ferocious hurricane. Mighty seas running free in the broad Atlantic struck the coast with indescribable force and filled the sky with spray and spume. The trawler *Big Cat*, Spanish built and registered in Falmouth, with a crew of fourteen mostly Spanish but with some British members, was running for shelter in Valentia harbour. Just as she was abeam of Cromwell's Point lighthouse her engines failed. Her mayday signal at 7.33 a.m. was intercepted by James Lynch on duty at Valentia Radio who immediately set the rescue machinery in motion.

Within minutes Paddy Gallagher had authorised the launch of the lifeboat and the *Margaret Frances Love* crewed by Coxswain Seanie Murphy, Mechanic Joseph

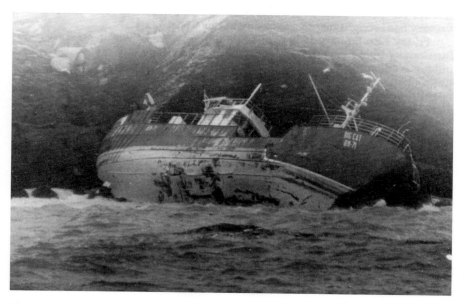

The wreck of the *Big Cat* on Beginish Island, 13 January 1989. Photo: John Cleary Photography, Tralee.

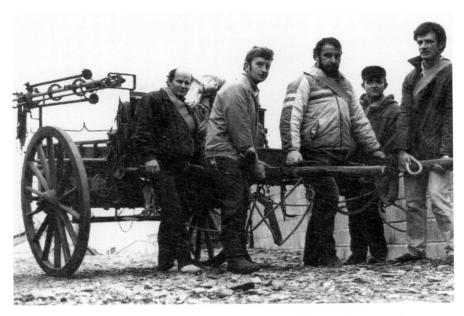

The *Rocket Car* which was transport provided for the Coast Lifesaving Service until early 1989. Crew members Donal Walsh, Peadar Houlihan, Aidan Walsh, Michael O'Connor and Owen Walsh. Left by the British, this is now on display in the Heritage Centre. Photo: John Cleary Photography, Tralee.

Houlihan, Assistant Mechanic Jimmy Murphy and crewmen Shane O'Neill, Tommy Gilligan and John Sheehan was racing to the scene.

They found the *Big Cat* aground on Beginish Island, stern first on the rocks and being washed from stem to stem by giant waves. Going alongside, veering down the lifeboat's inflatable dingy or operating a breeches buoy from the sea were all impossible. While air cover was requested from the Air Corps and RAF, the Coast Lifesaving Unit sprang into action. Michael O'Connor, Aidan Walsh, Owen Walsh, Pat Curtin and Peadar Houlihan were ferried with all the gear to Beginish Island by Donal Walsh in his fishing boat. All the gear had to be dragged over some 2 miles of rough ground to the scene of the wreck. The only assistance available was a wheelbarrow borrowed from Mike and Jim Casey. The two elderly men were the only inhabitants of the island. Later Aidan Linnane, Richard Quigley, Joseph O'Sullivan, Eamonn Murphy and Richard Foran together with some crew from a Spanish trawler joined the rescue team on Beginish.

Wet, cold and exhausted, again and again the rescuers sent their lifesaving breeches buoy down to the *Big Cat* and brought the frozen and frightened sailors to safety. It was only when Michael Shiel of Edinburgh was hauled ashore that it was learned that three had either been swept overboard or were trapped in the engine room. The lifeboat immediately began to comb the sea around the wreck. As soon as the Air Corps and RAF helicopters arrived they were asked by the lifeboat coxswain to fly the survivors to Caherciveen Hospital. This being done, an RAF diver was lowered to the wreck and confirmed that nobody was on board. The lifeboat recovered one body, wearing a lifejacket. Unfortunately that device was fitted back to front and had pushed the head of the unfortunate deceased into the water rather than keeping it out. Following this nine-hour service in savage conditions Coxswain Seanie Murphy received a framed letter of thanks from the Chairman of the RNLI for his seamanship and leadership. Mechanic Joseph Houlihan, Assistant Mechanic James Murphy and Lifeboatman John Sheehan received letters of thanks from the Chief of Operations. The director wrote to the members of the Coast Lifesaving Service Unit. The skill of the coxswain in co-ordinating the rescue was highly commended and praised by all concerned. In July 1992, 'Comhairle Na Mire Gaile', the Governments Official awards for bravery at sea, were presented at Caherciveen District Court. Justice Humphrey Kelleher presented the awards to Area Officer Micheal O'Connor, Pat Curtin, Owen Walsh, Peadar Houlihan and Aidan Walsh.

Aground on the Perch

On 1 December 1989 the fishing vessel *Westerly* of Dublin went aground on the Perch Rock in Valentia harbour. The weather was calm and there was good visibility. The lifeboat *Margaret Frances Love* slipped moorings at 7.25 p.m., with Second Coxswain Richard Connolly in charge. The boarding boat was taken in tow. Efforts were made to get the trawler off the rock. At 10.45 p.m. the Skipper asked that the crew be taken off as the trawler was listing dangerously. Manned by Andrew Quigley and Nealie Lyne the boarding boat transferred first ten and then the other six crew to the lifeboat. All sixteen were landed at Valentia pier. At high water a local boat put the crew back on board the *Westerly* at high tide and she sailed off.

In 1990 the lifeboat launched ten times sample services were as follows:

Valentia one of Eleven Lifeboats at Sea in Violent Storm

The 25 January 1990 was a day of ferocious storm. It crossed all coasts of Great Britain and Ireland. Lifeboats were launched at Lerwick, Barra Island, Eyemouth, Newcastle, Co. Down, Whitby, Flamborough, Bridlington, Lowestoft, Gorleston and Newhaven as well as Valentia.

The fishing vessel *Stella Orion* of Fleetwood had an injured man on board. She was 12 miles west of the Great Blasket Island in a north-westerly storm of force ten. The lifeboat crew assembled. When lift off by helicopter proved impossible, there was a grave danger of further injury to the patient. By link call, Coxswain Seanie Murphy arranged with the skipper to bring his vessel into Valentia harbour. Here she rendezvoused with the *Margaret Frances Love*. Dr Alan O Sullivan was put on board the trawler. The casualty was transferred to the lifeboat and landed at Renard pier.

Worst Night in Living Memory

Less than a week later the lifeboat was called again. On Tuesday 30 January word was received that the British-registered fishing vessel *Garadoza* was aground on rocks between Roancarrig More and Roancarrig beg in Bantry Bay. The *Kerryman* of 2 February 1990 described the service by the *Margaret Frances Love*.

> Valentia Boat's 'Worst Night in Memory'
> The Valentia Lifeboat struggled through sixty-foot waves off the Skellig Rock on Tuesday night to come to the assistance of a Spanish Trawler in whose rescue Irish Navy Man Michael Quinn perished. Secretary of the Valentia Lifeboat, Paddy Gallagher, said it was one of the worst nights in memory that the Valentia lifeboat took to the sea to become involved in a rescue. Seas were so rough that the lifeboat, under Coxswain Seanie Murphy took three hours and ten minutes to come to the Spanish Trawler which had run aground. The journey would normally take one hour and 45 minutes. 'The young leading seaman who lost his life was Michael Quinn of Ship Street, Drogheda and the Army Press Office denied reports that there was difficulty with VHF radio of the Command Ship on the scene, the L.E. *Deirdre*. The Crew of the *Garadoza* were airlifted by an RAF Helicopter. The seas were described as 'Phenomenal' at the time.

Casualty Washed Ashore

On 13 October 1990 the *Margaret Frances Love* launched into very high seas and a force ten south-easterly storm. A 10 foot rowing boat was reported drifting in Lough Kay. As the lifeboat reached the search area in atrocious conditions the casualty was taken by a massive wave and landed high on the rocks. The sole occupant was able to walk ashore.

Early in 1991 the RNLI announced that a new boathouse would be built at Valentia. At the same time Paddy Gallagher was awarded the Gold Badge by the RNLI in recognition of his long service.

In that year of 1991 the lifeboat launched nineteen times.

A Hopeless Dawn

On 9 March 1991 a call was received that a car had gone over a cliff at the Slea Head Area. In moderate sea the *Margaret Frances Love* reached the area. The car was at the waters edge. The Y boat was launched manned by Tommy Gilligan and Richard Quigley. With the assistance of the Gardaí and the Fire Brigade the bodies were transferred to the lifeboat and were landed at Dingle. The victims were aged seventeen, eighteen and twenty-one. This was a harrowing experience for the lifeboat men and all involved. It was devastating one for families, friends and indeed all west Kerry. In the *Irish Independent* of the 11 March 1991 Station Honorary Secretary Paddy Gallagher called for the provision of marine band radios at key Garda Stations. These could help the Gardaí to rapidly pinpoint emergency situations for lifeboat crews.

Yacht Escorted in Sixteen Hour Service

On 11 July 1991 in poor weather and rough seas the *Margaret Frances Love* launched at 2.40 a.m. They were responding to a call for assistance from the yacht *Squirrel* of Galway which had a medical emergency on board. The yacht was believed to be south of the Bull Rock. At 3.30 a.m. the Danish tall ship *Zenobegrammnoe* reported that she had located the yacht some 30 miles south-west of Castletownbere. At 5.15 a.m. a helicopter lifted the patient. At 6.35 a.m. the lifeboat reached the yacht which was then 24 miles south-west of Mizen Head. The yacht with the remaining two crew was escorted to Castletownbere harbour. After a meal the lifeboat returned to Valentia after some sixteen hours at sea.

Rosebud Towed in

On 13 September 1991 in rough seas and south-westerly wind force six to eight the fishing boat *Rosebud* of Tralee suffered engine failure. She was ¾ mile north of Coonanna harbour with two on board. The *Margaret Frances Love* slipped moorings at 7.15 p.m. and reached the casualty at 7.55 p.m. A rope was put on board and the casualty was saved and the two crew members rescued. She was towed to Caherciveen pier.

Wings of the Morning Towed for Twenty-Nine Miles

Two other lives were saved by the lifeboat *Margaret Frances Love* in 1991. On 29 October 1991 the American Yacht *Wings of the Morning* was storm battered and her rigging in tatters. She was 29 miles distant from Valentia, at 51.47 north 11.03 west, with two people on board. The weather and visibility were poor, seas were rough and there were 8 metre swells. The wind was south-south-west force eight when the lifeboat reached the casualty at 6.55 a.m. A tow line was put on board and the yacht was towed to safety and her two crew members rescued.

Wings of the Morning Towed in Again

The final service by the lifeboat for 1991 was on the 4 December. The *Wings of the Morning* was again in difficulty at 52.23 north 10.29 west 29 miles from station. She had engine failure and could not sail. There was a moderate sea and poor visibility. Leaving the moorings at 9 p.m. in a moderate sea the *Margaret Frances Love* reached the casualty at 11.18 p.m. and took her in tow to Valentia pier.

In 1992 there were ten launches.

Sailing Vessel with Broken Rudder Saved

On 2 May 1992 a small sailing dingy *Blue Sail* with three on board suffered a broken rudder ½ a mile west of Cromwell's Point lighthouse. She was heading for the rocks on Beginish Island adjacent to the lighthouse. The lifeboat *Duke of Atholl* was launched at 5.45 p.m. and reached the casualty at 5.50 p.m. The three people were taken on board the lifeboat and the dingy was towed to Caherciveen pier.

Three Canoes Were Safe

On 10 May 1992, the Gardaí at Dingle reported that six English tourists using three canoes had set out from the Minard Area. They had not returned to the Guest House, their cars were at the pier and there were fears for their safety. The lifeboat *Duke of Atholl* as well as an Air Corps helicopter combed the area from Kells to Slea head. Neither the helicopter nor the lifeboat located the casualties. The Dingle Gardaí later reported that the occupants of the canoes had come ashore and were camping in a field inside the harbour at Dingle.

Fishing Machine Rescued

On 22 July 1992 in south-west to west wind force five to six and a four-meter swell the *Fishing Machine* suffered engine failure. She was south of Doulous Head and drifting towards the nearby rocks.

She had a crew of three. The lifeboat *Margaret Frances Love* with Second Coxswain Richard Connolly in charge launched at 12.20 p.m. She reached the casualty at 1.30 p.m. A tow line was passed across and the casualty was towed to Valentia pier.

The owners treated the lifeboat crew to a dinner at a local restaurant.

On 21 August 1992 the Taoiseach Mr Albert Reynolds was brought by lifeboat from Caherciveen to Valentia. During the course of the visit he announced funding for a new slipway near the lifeboat store.

Joseph Houlihans Last 'Call Out'

On 18 December, Valentia Radio informed the Honorary Secretary Mr Gallagher that a Spanish fishing vessel was aground at Laght Point. This was the *Monti-Marie* with a crew of fourteen. The sea was calm and the weather was fine. The lifeboat *Margaret Frances Love* slipped moorings at 2.35 a.m. and was with the casualty at 2.45 a.m. It was feared the boat might capsize with the lowering tide as she was up on rocks. Six members of the crew were transferred by zodiac to the lifeboat. The lifeboat was joined by the fishing vessel *Spailpin Fanach* at 4 a.m. At 8.08 a.m. both vessels succeeded in towing the trawler clear of the rocks and she steamed to Renard Point.

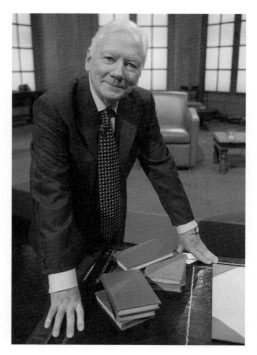

Gay Byrne, Ireland's greatest broadcaster presented the studio part of the 'Joe Houlihan Retirement Show'. Photo: courtesy of RTE.

This was Joseph Houlihan's last service on the Valentia lifeboat. As coincidence would have it, Joseph's first service was on the 26 November 1954 to the *Ros Airgead* ashore on the White Horse Rocks, a mere stone throw from Laght point. On 10 January 1993 the author wrote the following letter to *The Gay Byrne Show* then the most prestigious show in Irish Broadcasting:

Dear Gay,

On the 18th January 1993 Joseph Houlihan will retire from the position of mechanic of the Valentia Lifeboat. Could you please wish him, his wife Kathleen and family well for the future. This marks the end of a truly remarkable career in the lifeboat service.

Since he joined the lifeboat crew in 1954 there have been at least 300 service launches and at least 170 lives have been saved.

Joseph holds the Bronze Medal of the RNLI for bravery and has, on two occasions been awarded their thanks inscribed on vellum.

Medals and accolades, while always richly deserved are not the barometer of the dangers faced by the lifeboatmen. Because Valentia Harbour is the most Westerly harbour in Europe it gets the first harsh lash of the Atlantic Storms. The lifeboat there is farther out into the merciless ocean while still at her moorings than any other lifeboat in the entire fleet.

No lives were saved in some services undertaken in blood curdling conditions. The Christmas that the *Sea Flower* was lost the seas off the wild Kerry Coats were such that the lifeboat, at least once, heeled beyond the mathematical capsize point, but righted herself. Sixty-foot seas were encountered off the Skelligs on the occasion that the *Gardoza* was in trouble. (That was the occasion when a young Navy sailor was lost). So bad were the conditions when the *Capo Emma* called for assistance that some of those heroic lifeboat women were at the boathouse, in tears, when it appeared that conditions were too severe. Satisfied that the boat was up to the job the lifeboat launched. On those horrific nights and on many more, their seafaring skills and the Good Lord, as he is bid to do in Phil Coulters great anthem of the lifeboat service of the same name, brought them 'Home from the Sea'.

Add to this the horror of the Air India Crash 112 miles out from their station and the measuring of fuel, so as to give maximum search time, to bring them back to the Skelligs with almost dry tanks. The Keepers of the light provided the fuel to bring the five bodies of those tragic people the rest of the way to Valentia.

Personally, I believe that the spirit that motivates lifeboat people is of the soul. It is reinforced by the knowledge that people of the caliber of Joe Houlihan have their boat in all times at peak condition, no small factor when you take your lifebelt in the lifeboat store.

As well as local fishing and pleasure fleets Valentia Lifeboat has answered calls from vessels from Britain, France, Spain, Norway, Panama, Germany, Greece and the USA. The service Joseph has given to the seafaring community in his capacity as a lifeboatman transcends local and national boundaries. S0, I believe, does the debt of gratitude that follows such service.

Perhaps you might agree that a 'Thank You' over the airwaves, which transcend those very same boundaries, would be in order fro a man who has given such selfless service for so long in the cause of humanity.

Yours faithfully,

Richard J. Robinson.

The response was not that Gay would give a 'Thank You' over the air. It was a phone call to say the show would be presented from Valentia Lifeboat Station. Joe Houlihan was no man for fuss he would slip away quietly when he had said 'Finished with the engines' for the last time. So he retired live on RTE's *Gay Byrne Show* live on Radio 1.

When 'Tico's Tune', played by Manuel, hit the airwaves heralding the show on 26 January 1993 the million listeners heard Joe Duffy interview Joe Houlihan. Then, for the last time, Joe Houlihan brought the two great engines of the lifeboat *Margaret Frances Love* roaring to life near Cromwell's Point and the lifeboat returned to the pier. The programme was broadcast from the old lifeboat house. If even one amongst that million begrudged the accolade then they deserved to be left in splendid isolation. The show was Gay said not just a tribute to Joe but to all the lifeboat people who were notg half thanked nor appreciated enough.

Joe, his wife, Kathleen, sisters Derarca and Bridie and brother Pat were all interviewed by Joe Duffy. Pat was a surprise guest home from Scotland after 10 years. Coxswain Seanie Murphy told of how a balloon bursting had him out of bed and waiting for the second maroon to launch the boat. Ex-Coxswain Dermot Walsh recalled the "Oranmore" rescue and produced the letter he had received from the widow of Mr. Lennon who died of a heart attack during the operation. He also told of relieving workmen in Inisvickillane and how Mr Haughey had sent a case of rum to the crew and had continued to do so. Ex-Second Coxswain Des Lavelle recalled the horrendous conditions encountered on the *Sea Flower* rescue, Station Historian Dick Robinson, filled in with historical pieces as required by Joe Duffy. He told the story of the Baltimore lifeboatman who allegedly asked Mr Haughey, whom they had rescued for a state funeral. This on the basis that the crewmember's father would kill him when he learned who they had rescued. Leo Houlihan, newly appointed mechanic told of the recovery of three bodies from near Dingle when a car went over a cliff on what he described as 'A Black Day'. Telephone link ups were made with Delores O'Connor in Milton Keynes who had been rescued by the lifeboat. Eamon De Buitlear also told of being rescued by Valentia lifeboat when he and a party of ornithologists were marooned on the Great Blasket Island. Kieran Cotter Bronze Medalist coxswain of Baltimore lifeboat called and told of his medal rescue. Former Taoiseach Charles Haughey

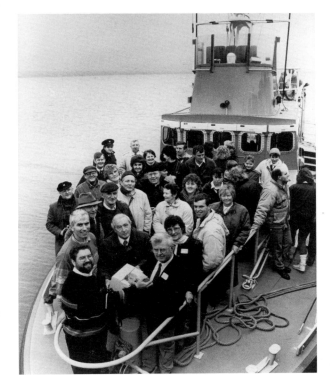

Right: Joe Duffy makes
a presentation to Joe
Houlihan. Photo: Dick
Robinson Collection.

Below: Phil Coulter and
guests on Valentia Lifeboat
after *The Gay Byrne Show*.
Photo: Dick Robinson
Collection.

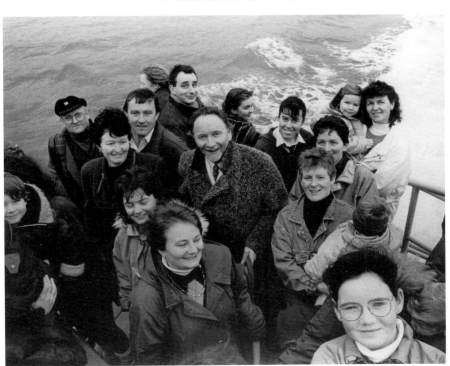

joined in the conversation. With praise of the crews and recalled his rescue at Mizen Head. Phil Coulter had been asked to take a phone call but decided to come in person and told his story. The sea had brought tragedy to his family on two occasions. As a result he had come into contact with the RNLI and wrote the great anthem of the lifeboat service 'Home from the Sea' which he performed. The local folk group led by Fr P.J. O Sullivan joined in with talented relish. Musicians Dan Mc Crohen, Mary Gallagher, Kevin Larkin and Russel Orpen also entertained.

Valentia Radio was always on hand to keep in touch, their advice that Joe Duffy be thrown overboard was not accepted. Station Secretary Paddy Gallagher had given every assistance with the show. Martin Moriarty fired maroons. Joe was presented with Waterford Glass on behalf of the crew. In wrapping up the show Gay Byrne said that in honouring Joe Houlihan they were also honouring all lifeboat people everywhere.

At the end of the show it fell to the author to salute the lifeboat service: Joe Duffy: 'Salute the Lifeboats, Dick Robinson'.

The people who give without any thought for themselves. They go to sea without any hope for reward, I think it is the highest possible motivation. It is a code of the sea. It has been as long as the sea has been there, it will be as long as the sea will be there and we are proud to be part of it. We are proud of Joe Houlihan, of all who served of all who have served and those who went before us we remember them with tremendous pride and affection. Those who serve everywhere WE SALUTE THEM.

The back up team from RTE who travelled to Valentia was: producer Ronan Kelly, broadcasting assistant Ann Farrell and outside broadcasting men Johnny Culloty and Johnny Craig.

Joe Houlihan had been awarded the Bronze Medal of the RNLI. At 6.55 a.m. on the evening of 2 September 1963, lifeboat mechanic Joseph Houlihan was working at the lifeboat store. He saw a small dinghy capsize about 600 yards away. The sea was very rough with a near gale blowing from the north. The weather was fine and clear. It was an hour and a half after high water on an exceptionally high spring tide. The tide was ebbing at two knots. Singlehanded, he immediately launched the 12 foot 6 inch boarding boat and rowed to the capsized dinghy which was 200 yards from Reenagiveen point. He found two men in the water, one virtually collapsed. The other man, a clergyman, was too heavy to pull on board. The man on board could be of no assistance as he was exhausted. Joe instructed the second survivor to hold the transom of the boat and he rowed to shore towing the hapless clergyman behind. In a following sea and with the boat trimming by the stern this was a most difficult operation and Joe was practically exhausted himself when he reached shore. For this rescue Joe was awarded the

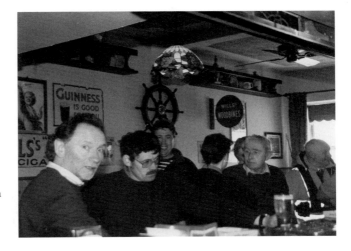

Phil Coulter in Boston's Bar with Valentia lifeboat crew on 3 May 1996, following a concert in Ennis the previous night. Ralph and Nana McTell accompanied him. Photo: Dick Robinson.

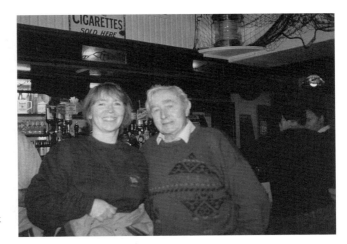

Nana McTell and Paddy Gallagher, 3 May 1996. Photo: Dick Robinson.

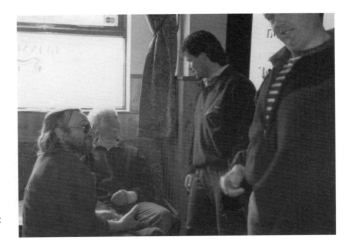

Martin Moriarty, Seanie Murphy (coxswain), Richard Quigley and D. Gallagher at Bostons on 3 May 1996. Photo: Dick Robinson.

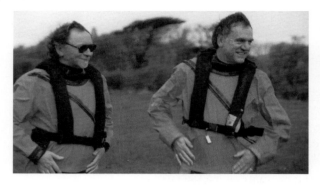

Phil Coulter and Ralph Mc
Tell after alighting from the
Sea Rescue Helicopter at
Valentia on 3 May 1996.
They were visiting Valentia
Lifeboat.

Bronze Medal, making him the first Valentia lifeboat man to receive an RNLI medal. There was a follow-up to this incident. In their book *Strong to Save* Ray and Susannah Kipling tell the story:

> Eagle-eyed officials at R.N.L.I. headquarters in London spotted a gap in a report from Valentia. The machinery log showed that the mechanic had been absent for four days and no explanation had been given. A polite letter was sent to the honorary secretary, who must have taken great delight in sending the following reply: 'I acknowledge receipt of your letter re Mechanic J. Houlihan being absent from 4th to 9th April. Houlihan was attending the Annual General Meeting in London where he received the award of the Institution's Bronze Medal.'

Another individual rescue was to bring Joe the thanks of the RNLI inscribed on vellum.

At 11.19 a.m. on 26 August 1982, Valentia Coast Radio Station made a general broadcast requesting assistance for an angler who had been washed off the rocks at Culloo Head. Joe Houlihan, who was on leave from his lifeboat duties, was demonstrating a Fastworker boat to a potential customer at the 'Coastguard Patch'. He intercepted the call on VHF. There was a gale-force six wind gusting to force seven from the west and a very rough sea.

Driving the Fastworker at best speed, Joseph arrived off the cliffs at 11.40 a.m. There onlookers directed him to the casualty. There was a considerable backwash and seas were 5 to 6 metres high. The boat was brought alongside the casualty and the angler was brought on board. Having cleared the dangerous shoreline the boat was stopped and Joseph satisfied himself that the man was alright and provided him with warm clothing. Valentia lifeboat, which was on the way to the scene was recalled and the angler was landed into the care of a doctor and an ambulance at Reenard Point. Letters of appreciation from the RNLI were sent to Michael O'Connor, the crewman and John O'Connor, the potential Fastworker customer, recording their part in the rescue. Joe had served as second coxswain/mechanic in 1977.

Two Consecutive Services

On 28 April 1993 RNLB *Margaret Frances Love* was launched at 7.20 p.m. to the assistance of the local fishing vessel *Béal Bocht*, which had suffered engine failure 300 yards west of the Small Skelligs Rock.

There were four people on board. The vessel was taken in tow to Portmagee pier. On arrival at Portmagee, the lifeboat was informed that the fishing vessel *Prospective* needed assistance at 52.23 north and 10.29 west. She set off immediately. The casualty was taken in tow at 12.25 a.m. and towed to Dingle. The lifeboat was back at moorings at 6 a.m. after a long night.

Injured Lady Taken off Skelligs

On 19 May 1993, a lady was injured while visiting the Skelligs Rock. The *Margaret Frances Love* slipped mooring at 5 p.m. and arrived at the rock at 5.50 p.m. There was a swell and strong currents at the landing stage at the Skelligs. Coxswain Murphy held the lifeboat offshore. Assistant Mechanic Martin Moriarty went ashore in the Y boat. The casualty was placed in a stretcher and brought to the lifeboat.

Her husband and a friend were also taken on board. First aid was given by the coxswain and assistant mechanic. The casualty was landed into the care of an ambulance crew at Renard Point. During 1993 the floor of the 1864 boathouse was removed at Renard Point. There is now a car park on the site.

Three Casualties in High Seas

On 1 August 1993, foul weather made Dingle Bay a very unfriendly place. A south-westerly wind force seven to eight was blowing, the seas were very high and there were 4 metre swells. Both the weather and the visibility were poor. At 5.35 p.m. Valentia Radio contacted Mr Gallagher to state that the French yacht *Les Bibes* needed assistance in adverse conditions.

The *Margaret Frances Love* slipped moorings at 5.50 p.m. Arriving at the casualty at 6.30 p.m, Coxswain Murphy asked the *Fionan of Skellig* to take the yacht in tow as there were now two other casualties to be dealt with. The lifeboat proceeded to a 26 foot pleasure boat with three on board which was in danger of being blown ashore due to a fouled propeller. The lifeboat connected a tow line and towed the vessel to Kells. Immediately then began to search for the third vessel. This was a small fishing boat with three people on board. She was sighted at 10.50 a.m. and escorted to safe harbour at Kells. Mr Gallagher in his remarks stated, 'This was a most unusual service as three very good services were carried out in adverse weather conditions in a very competent manner'.

Twelve-Hour Service in Tough Conditions

The Spanish fishing vessel *Dumnovia* suffered engine failure on 12 September 1993. She was 4 miles south-west of the Bull Rock with a crew of twelve on board. The wind was east-north-east force six to eight and the sea was very rough. There were 3 metre swells.

The *Margaret Frances Love* slipped moorings at 7.25 a.m. with second coxswain Richard Connolly in charge. The casualty was reached at 9.15 a.m. and a tow line was connected. The trawler was towed to Castletownbere. A hot meal was provided for the lifeboat crew. The lifeboat was refuelled and ready for service at 7.10 p.m. after almost twelve hours at sea in tough conditions.

Ocean Wanderer Towed in

The *Ocean Wanderer*, with a crew of three, was one mile off the land, north of Valentia, on 5 October 1993 when her propeller was fouled. Seas were very rough and the wind was north-easterly force six to eight. The *Margaret Frances Love* launched at 10.05 a.m. with Second Coxswain Richard Connolly in charge. She reached the casualty at 10.25 a.m. and a tow line was put on board. She was towed to Valentia pier.

In 1994, Valentia lifeboat launched fourteen times including the services hereunder:

Off the Moorings in Five Minutes

A north-westerly wind force six to eight was blowing and seas were very rough on 7 July 1994. The trawler *Marber Therese*, with a crew of four fouled her propeller 2 miles north of Reenadrolane Point (The Wireless Point). At 7.05 p.m. just five minutes after the signal was received the lifeboat Hibernia under coxswain Seanie Murphy slipped moorings. Arriving at the casualty at 7.35 p.m a tow line was established with some difficulty. The Trawler and her four crew were safely landed at Portmagee.

Helping Mary Harper

There is always something different on the sea. The 7 August 1994 was a beautiful day. Seas were calm, a north-easterly breeze force three to four was blowing and the weather and visibility was good. Nevertheless at 2.30 p.m. a call came from the Canadian flagged yacht *Quan Ying 2* of Boston that she had suffered engine failure. She was 30 miles south-west of Valentia. She had a fuel shortage. Under Second Coxswain Richard Connolly the *Hibernia* embarked twenty gallons of fuel. She then set off for the casualty area. They reached the *Quan Ying 2* at 5.30 p.m. They found the sole crew member exhausted. The lifeboat crew helped to refuel and clean up the yacht.

Despite being tired and weary the yachtswoman, seventy-nine-year-old Mary Harper, who had sailed single-handed from Boston, insisted on carrying on her journey under power to Crookhaven. On being satisfied that all was now well the lifeboat returned to station. Ms Harper made a donation of $200 to the station.

Bad Weather Escort for *Dotty Dee*

Exactly one month later, on the 7 September 1994, another Canadian yacht was in distress off the Kerry Coast. The *Dotty Dee*, with a crew of two, had a broken mast. She was in rough seas and a force six south-westerly wind with 3 metre swells. *Hibernia* slipped moorings at 12.25 a.m. and reached the casualty at 1.10 a.m. The mast and sailings were hanging off the vessel. Coxswain Murphy passed cutters across to the owner of the yacht. After cutting the stays and tidying up the yacht proceeded to Valentia escorted by the lifeboat.

Trawler Saved at Inis Nabro

On 14 September 1994, the lifeboat *Hibernia* responded to a distress call from the trawler *Straithnair*. The trawler with a crew of five was in danger of going aground on Inis Nabro in the Blasket Islands. The lifeboat reached the casualty at 11.15 p.m. and put a tow line on board. The casualty was towed south out of danger. The Dingle trawler *Thanet J* arrived on the scene and took the rescued trawler in tow to Dingle. The 1946 lifeboat store was demolished in January 1994. The roof was removed on the 14 January and the rest was bulldozed on the 16 January 1995. Replica Roundels were included in the new building.

In 1995 the Valentia lifeboat crew assembled nineteen times and launched eighteen times including the services recorded hereunder:

Assistance for Boat and Nine Divers

On 3 June 1995 the honorary secretary, Mr Gallagher, received a message from Valentia Radio. There was a semi-rigid inflatable with nine divers on board in difficulties. She was understood to be south of Puffin Island. The *Margaret Frances Love* slipped moorings at 5.35 p.m. and headed for the casualty area. The vessel was unsure of her position. At 5.45 p.m. the coxswain was informed that Cuas

Crom was the position. Coxswain Murphy established the position by VHF/DF.
The casualty was reached at 6 p.m. Seven of the divers were taken on board the
lifeboat and the inflatable taken in tow to Knightstown pier.

Thirty-Seven and a Half-Mile Tow for Trawler

On 25 July 1995, the *Jemaleen* of Cork lost her steering. She was 37½ miles north-
north-west of Valentia. The *Margaret Frances Love* slipped her moorings at 10.25
p.m. The weather was good and seas were slight. Wind was south-easterly force
five. She reached the casualty at 12.55 a.m. A tow line was connected and the
trawler was towed to Valentia. The lifeboat was refuelled and ready for service at
7 a.m. on 26 July.

Fire on the Skelligs Rock

On 26 July 1995 a serious situation arose on the Great Skellig Rock. A fire had
taken hold and huts used by Office of Public Works staff were ablaze. Gas cylin-
ders used for heating and cooking were heating and exploding.

The *Margaret Frances Love* slipped moorings at 5.05 p.m. in calm weather and
good visibility. She reached the rock at 6.10 p.m. Seven workers shaken but not
seriously injured were taken onboard the lifeboat and were landed at Valentia
(Knightstown pier).

In 1996, there were twenty-seven launches by the Valentia lifeboat. These included
the following services:

Time up for 52-23

On 28 August 1996 the fishing vessel *Ocean Wanderer* fouled her propeller a mile
off the shore north of Valentia. Wind was north-westerly force four and seas were
moderate. The *Margaret Frances Love* slipped moorings at 7.02 p.m. She reached
the casualty at 7.17 p.m. and towed her with her two crew on board to Knights
town pier. This was the final service performed at Valentia Bay by the *Margaret
Frances Love*

At Valentia she had launched 192 times and saved seventy-three lives. She was
assigned to Barry Dock Station in South Wales from May 1997 to August 2003.
Here she launched on service 129 times and saved ten lives. As at the end of
December 2008 she was named *Huaying 398* and is currently serving as a lifeboat
at Donghoi, Shanghai, China.

NINE

A NEW SEVERN CLASS LIFEBOAT – *JOHN & MARGARET DOIG*

On 30 October 1996, a new Severn class lifeboat arrived at Valentia. RNLB *John and Margaret Doig* (ON1218) (17-07) was escorted into harbour by the RNLB *Margaret Frances Love* and berthed at Knightstown Quay 3.30 p.m. She had encountered some appalling weather on the passage and had acquitted herself well. The boat was provided from a legacy of Miss Mary Doig together with other legacies. The hull was built by Green Marine Ltd and the boat was fitted out at FBM Ltd in Cowes. The cost of the boat was £1,580,000 (sterling). She is powered by two 1,250 horse-power Caterpillar diesel engines. District Inspector Colin Williams was in charge for the passage.

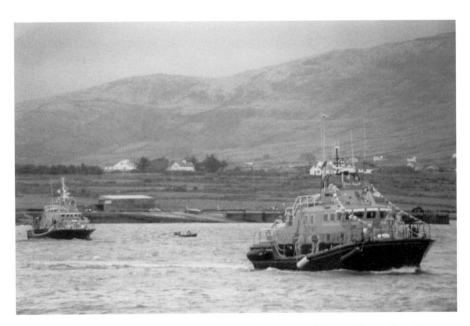

O.N.1218 The *John and Margaret Doig* escorted in by O.N. 1082 *Margaret Frances Love*. Photo: Dick Robinson.

Valentia Lifeboats: A History

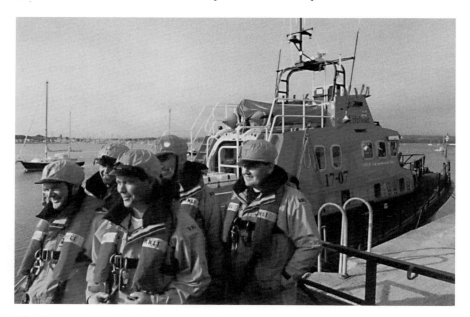

Valentia crew training at Poole. Front row, from left to right: Conn O' Shea and Richard Quigley. Back row: Junior Murphy, Seanie Murphy and Leo Houlihan, 2006. Photo: courtesy of Tony Denton.

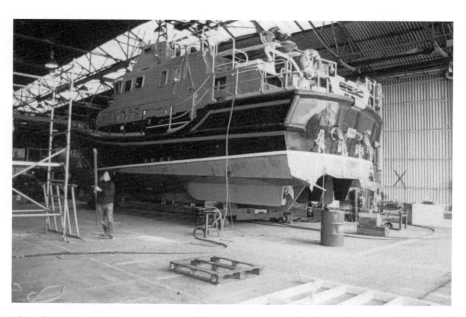

The *John and Margaret Doig* at Souters, 15 January 1996. Photo: courtesy of Tony Denton.

First Call for New Severn Class Lifeboat

On 18 November 1996, the new Severn class lifeboat *John and Margaret Doig* (ON 1218) answered her first service call.

The dredger *Germaine* of Arklow, with seven people on board was dragging her anchor in Valentia harbour. She was in danger of going ashore. The weather was appalling at the time. There was a south-easterly wind force nine blowing. Seas were very rough and swell of 4 metres within the harbour. Mechanic Leo Houlihan and District Engineer Ireland Derek Potter were on board the lifeboat when the call was received. Slipping her moorings at 8.50 p.m. Coxswain Murphy decided that the best course of action was to escort the dredger to Caherciveen. This was done and the lifeboat returned to station at 10.15 p.m.

French Fishing Vessel with Nine Crew Saved

The new lifeboat performed her first lifesaving service on 3 December 1996. Atrocious weather conditions pertained at the time. North-westerly wind force nine, very rough seas and 5 to 7 metre swells and only fair visibility was the mix.

At 3.35 p.m. the assembly signal was made and at 3.45 p.m the *John and Margaret Doig* slipped moorings. The casualty was the French fishing vessel *Tourmalet* of Concarneau with a crew of nine on board. She had had a net in the propeller and was fearful of being driven aground on the Foze Rock.

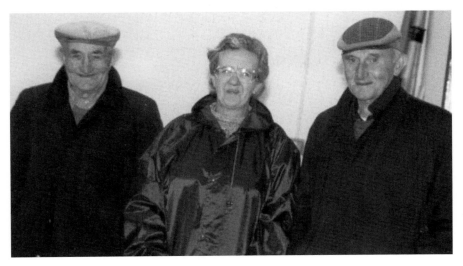

Waiting for the Severn. Miko Leary, former crew, Tess Robinson, Ennis Fundraising Branch and Dodie Walsh former second coxswain. Photo: Dick Robinson.

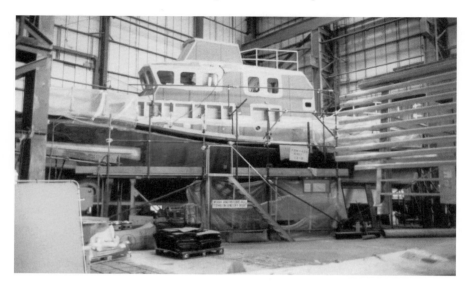

Valentia lifeboat in build at Souters on 23 August 1995. Fairey builders rented space from Souters. Photo: courtesy of Tony Denton.

The lifeboat reached the casualty at 5 p.m. After some difficulty, a tow rope was put on board. The vessel was towed to Dingle. Given the conditions, the tow proceeded at three to three and a half knots. The lifeboat left Dingle at 1 a.m. and returned to station.

In 1997 the Valentia lifeboat launched on thirty-two occasions including the following:

Two Saved in Rough Weather

On 23 April 1997, the fishing vessel *Skellig Dawn* suffered engine failure in the Blaskets Area. With a crew of two she was between Inisvickillane and Inish Nabro. The sea was rough with 3 to 4 metre swells. The *John and Margaret Doig* slipped moorings as 12.52 p.m. and reached the casualty at 1.32 p.m. A tow line was put on board and the saved craft and her rescued crew were brought safely to Valentia harbour.

Body Found After Night Search

On 13 June 1997, Mr Gallagher received a telephone message at 11.20 that Mr James Courtney of Caherciveen, in an 18 foot boat with an outboard engine, had not returned to Caherciveen. His relatives were concerned for his safety. At 11.25 p.m. the *John and Margaret Doig* slipped her moorings. The crew was already in the vicinity of the station, preparing for the naming ceremony the following day. It was a calm night with good visibility. A thorough search was made around Doulus Head and north of Valentia. At 4.30 a.m. Coxswain Murphy decided to launch the Y boat to search the caves. The Y boat, manned by Andrew Quigley and Con O'Shea located the boat in the Cathedral Cave some 100 metres from the entrance. At 5.15 a.m. the body was of the man was located in 8 feet of water and was recovered. It was transferred to the lifeboat and landed at Renard pier to the waiting ambulance.

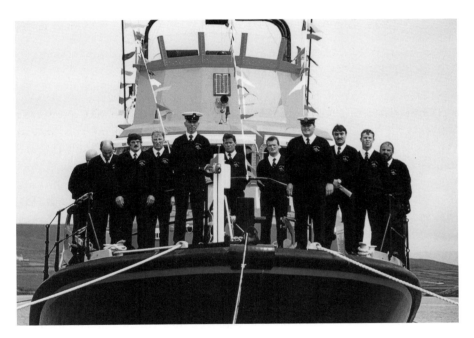

Valentia crew at the naming ceremony. Photo: Dick Robinson.

The Naming Ceremony, 14 June 1997

The day of the ceremony itself was beautiful. The lifeboat was anchored off the new boarding boat slipway, adjacent to the new station. After the National Anthem, Revd Fr John Shanahan, chairman of the Valentia Branch welcomed the guests and opened the proceedings. Mr Clayton Love Jr Deputy Chairman of the

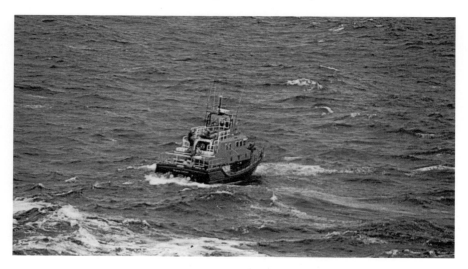

The lifeboat with two German survivors and a body on board searching off Culloo Head for a fourth person washed off the rocks. Photo: Dick Robinson.

RNLI opened the new boathouse. Mr Colin Williams, Inspector of Lifeboats in Ireland, described the lifeboat. Mr Richard Dixon representing the donors delivered the lifeboat to the RNLI. Mr Clayton Love Jnr accepted the lifeboat and delivered it into the care of Valentia Lifeboat Station. Mr Paddy Gallagher, station honorary secretary accepted the lifeboat. Bishop Bill Murphy and Bishop Edward Darling performed the service of dedication with hymns by the local Choir. Mr Tim Lyne, deputy launching authority, proposed the vote of thanks. Mr Charles J. Haughey, Former Taoiseach, named the lifeboat. The lifeboat put to sea with the platform party and guests on board. The gathering was a great event. Irish RNLI personnel were Anne Sweeney, Anna Classan, Angus Watson and Claire Brennan as well as Mr Williams. Virtually all stations were represented. Lt Commander George Cooper and Michael Vlasto attended from Poole. Mr Jim Wallbridge from London attended his 176th naming ceremony and lifeboat enthusiast Tony Denton with his wife Maureen from Shrewsbury were also in attendance.

Two Saved at Culoo

On 30 July 1997, the honorary secretary received a phone call from Mr John J. O'Connor that four people had been washed off the rocks at Culloo and needed immediate assistance. At 3.09 p.m., seven minutes after the call was received the *John and Margaret Doig* slipped her moorings. At 3.23 p.m. the lifeboat reached the search area in heavy seas and big ground swell. A lifebuoy and heaving line had already been prepared. On arrival, two survivors were seen in the water just outside the surf line. Coxswain Sean Murphy positioned the lifeboat so that the buoy and heaving line would reach the survivors. Once they had taken hold of the buoy the lifeboat was brought slowly astern out of the danger area and away from the rocks. The two survivors were brought aboard. In order to facilitate this crew member Andrew Quigley was lowered over the side wearing a safety harness. The survivors were given first aid and wrapped in blankets.

Ned Carey from Kilcummin in Killarney was alive when he was taken from the water. First Aid was administered but the victim failed to respond. A medical person was lowered from the Rescue Helicopter and confirmed that the man was dead. The search for the fourth person continued until the light faded.

The survivors, German ladies Dorothea Satter and Beatrex Kolb, were taken to Tralee General Hospital where they made a full recovery. Four days later the body of twenty-nine-year-old Paul Elliott was recovered by Naval and Garda Divers.

There was universal praise for the lifeboat crew and their efforts. The speed and stability of the Severn class lifeboat were also factors. Coxswain Seanie Murphy was awarded a letter of thanks by the RNLI.

Water Pumped from Leaking Trawler

On 17 August 1997, at 9.42 p.m. Mr Gallagher was informed by Valentia Radio that the trawler *Castor et Pollux* needed assistance. The trawler was taking in water. She was at the mouth of Kenmare River some 17 miles from the station.

Eight minutes after the alarm was raised the RNLB *John and Margaret Doig* slipped her moorings. The casualty was reached at 10.47 p.m. The lifeboat came alongside and Mechanic Leo Houlihan and crewman Richard Quigley went on board taking a portable pump with them. They succeeded in pumping out water and starting the engine. The casualty was taken in tow to Portmagee pier. Two people were rescued in this service. There were a total of thirty-two launches of the Valentia lifeboat in 1997.

In 1998 Mr Gallagher was awarded a bar to his Gold Badge.

Rescue from the Rocks at Small Skelligs

On the 14 April 1998 Valentia Radio informed Mr Gallagher that the motor vessel *Thundercrest* was on the rocks at the Small Skelligs. The passengers were on the Rocks and the skipper was still on board the vessel. At 2 p.m. and seven minutes after the distress signal was received the lifeboat RNLB *John and Margaret Doig* slipped her moorings.

Arriving at the scene thirty-five minutes later in a moderate to choppy sea Coxswain Murphy saw people on the rocks with the vessel inside in Cuas, a small cave.

The coxswain immediately decided to launch the Y boat. Crew members Andrew and Richard Quigley were on board. They were instructed to evacuate the people two at a time. All nine passengers were brought on board the lifeboat. The skipper of the casualty was still on board and was unable to get out of the boat onto the rocks. Coxswain Murphy left mechanic Leo Houlihan in command of the lifeboat and boarded the Y Boat with the two crewmen.

On reaching the cave Coxswain Murphy realised that he could not reach the skipper due to the high seas. He got onto the rocks and got hold of the life-raft from the casualty which was floating in the area. He inflated the life-raft. Manoeuvring from the rocks, he passed the heaving line which was attached to the life-raft to the skipper on the casualty. It was then found that the canopy had to be cut off the life-raft to enable the skipper to get on board. The skipper of the casualty used the heaving line to bring the life-raft into the cave and got on board. The raft was then hauled out to the Y boat. He was taken to the vessel *Small Una* which was in the area. With all ten people rescued the lifeboat headed for home after a very successful rescue carried out with great efficiency and speed in dangerous conditions.

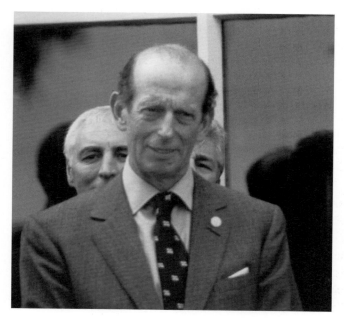

HRH The Duke of Kent -President of the RNLI - who visited Valentia Lifeboat Station on 5 June 1998. Photo: Dick Robinson.

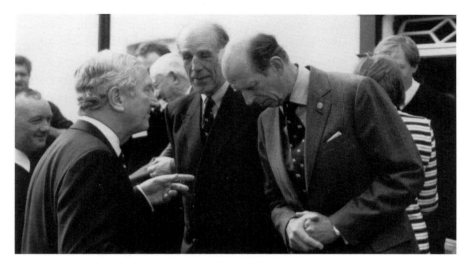

HRH The Duke of Kent (president) with Mr David Ackland (chairman) and Lieutenant Commander Brian Miles (director and secretary, RNLI). They visited Valentia Lifeboat Station on 5 June 1998. Photo: Dick Robinson.

Twelve Lives Saved in Eleven-Hour Service

On 22 April 1998 IMES in Dublin informed Mr Gallagher that the yacht *Army New Age* had a broken mast and steering problems. She was some 26 miles north-west of the station.

RNLB *John and Margaret Doig* slipped moorings at 4.40 p.m. with Second Coxswain Richard Connolly in command. The wind was south-westerly force five to seven and the sea was rough. The casualty valued at €250,000 and with a crew of twelve was located. She was taken in tow to Dingle the lifeboat then returning to station. The lifeboat had been at sea for nearly twelve hours. Twelve lives were saved.

'Valentia Rolls out Red Carpet for its Third Royal Visitor'

History was made in Valentia, Co. Kerry, yesterday [5 June 1988] when the island welcomed its third Royal visitor in 140 years.

The Duke of Kent, in his capacity as patron of the RNLI, helicoptered in to pay a courtesy call to the Valentia lifeboat and to honour a service that has helped save more than 700 lives off the Kerry Coast since the first lifeboat came to the island in 1865.

'I'm impressed with the warm welcome particularly from a small seaside place,' commented the Duke, who was formally greeted by Valentia Lifeboat

Secretary Paddy Gallagher and other officials. There was discreet Garda security for the visit, but only a handful of people, including locals and a few tourists were at the pier when the VIP helicopter touched down.

The Duke walked smartly to the lifeboat house where he met coxswain Seanie Murphy and the 16 strong local crew and had tea with them and dignitaries such as Kerry County Council Chairman Cllr. P.J. Cronin.

Valentia Parish Priest, Very Rev. John Shanahan, delved into the history books to trace royal connections with Valentia and found that Prince Albert Edward, son of Queen Victoria visited in 1858. Prince Arthur Patrick came to the island in 1869 and the Royal Hotel, Valentia was dedicated to him.

Prince Arthur Patrick visited the residence of the Knight of Kerry, here on the island, but had to call off a planned trip to the Skelligs Rock as the seas were too high and he was reputed to have been a bad sailor' stated Fr. Shanahan

The Priest also referred to close links between Valentia and England, pointing out that many English people were already in the area and many Irish people had found a welcome in England where they made their home.

'We get a lot of letters from people in England whose ancestors came from here' he told the Duke.

Also in the visiting party were The British Ambassador Veronica Sutherland, David Ackland, Chairman RNLI; Brian Miles, Director, RNLI and Clayton Love, Vice President. The Duke had also visited the Ballycotton lifeboat and travelled by car to Youghal where he met the crew members and fundraising committee. He spent over an hour with them and congratulates them on their work both fund-raising and lifesaving.

(That report from *The Examiner* of Saturday 6th June 1998. The Duke had also visited Courtmacsherry and Baltimore Lifeboat Stations.)

The *Kerryman* on 4 December 1998 profiled Valentia Lifeboat Station as the final nominee in the AIB/Kerryman Awards. Under the title 'The guardians of the south west coast' Nick Miller wrote:

The south west coast is reckoned to be the roughest in Ireland and the crew of the Valentia Lifeboat Station are regularly placed in life threatening situations. 'The area covered is very rough territory' says Honorary Secretary Paddy Gallagher.

They also have to undergo some fairly gruelling tasks. When an Air India aeroplane crashed 120 miles off Ireland the crew was enlisted to recover bodies.' It was like a battlefield at the time with bodies thrown all over the place' Paddy says.

Paddy was an Achill Island Man. He had retired from the position of Environmental Health Officer a year and a half before the awards. He came to Kerry fresh from College in 1956.

I got very involved in the GAA and married a local girl in 1962. Paddy's wife Joan (*née* Burke) was then principal of Scoil Deararca. They had six children.

Paddy was then the longest serving Lifeboat Secretary in the entire RNLI network.

'The lifeboat staff are very dedicated, they are very concerned about people' Paddy says 'There is a great tradition on the western seaboard amongst fishermen that if there is a boat in trouble they will try and save them. Most of these lads would have been involved in fishing and that is where the dedication comes from'. Although the crew is currently an all male affair, it did have a female member at one stage. Valentia Lifeboat was declared winners of the Merit Award 1988.

In 1999 there were sixteen launches of the Valentia lifeboat. Five lives were saved by Valentia lifeboat in 1999.

Yacht and Crew saved in Rough Seas

The yacht *Enterprise* of Kilrush had a broken mast. She was at position 52.03 north and 10.56 west and was 25.2 miles from the lifeboat station. There were five persons, four male and one female on board.

The lifeboat *John and Margaret Doig* slipped moorings at 7.40 a.m. and set out into rough seas. There was a force five to seven south-easterly wind. By the time the casualty was reached at 8.50 a.m. the wind had increased to force seven to nine south-easterly and the sea was very rough. A tow was established under difficult conditions and the slow tow to safe haven began. The casualty was towed into Valentia harbour at 5.30 p.m. and was taken to Caherciveen where she was secured alongside.

Sudden Death of Long Serving Honorary Secretary

On Sunday 18 July, while attending the Munster final in Cork, Paddy Gallagher died suddenly. Fulsome and deserving tributes were paid to him by the RNLI and the GAA. At Kerry County Council's next meeting, following tributes by Councillor O'Donoghue and Councillor Jackie Healy-Rae a vote of sympathy was supported by all members and a minutes silence was observed. Tributes were paid many other individuals and groups. Mr Richard Foran was appointed honorary secretary in September 1999.

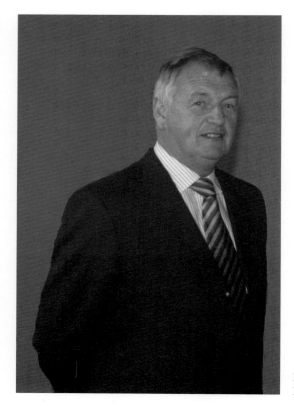

Richard Foran. Photo: courtesy of
Richard Foran.

In 2000 the lifeboat responded to twenty-five calls.

Man Dissuaded from Cliff Jump

At 10.55 a.m. on 11 June 2000 a member of the public advised the coxswain that
there was an incident developing at Culloo Cliffs. The coxswain advised honorary secretary Mr Foran. The *John and Margaret Doig* was launched and went to
the scene. On arrival they observed a young man standing at the verge of the
cliffs. He was in a very distressed state and threatening to jump. The lifeboat stood
by. Members of the public dissuaded him from jumping and the incident was
resolved at 11.30 a.m. the lifeboat returning to station.

Sick Fisherman Landed at Fenit

On 30 June 2000, the trawler *Ardent* had a crewman on board who had been
bleeding from the nose intermittently for some twenty-four hours. He had

refused an airlift and the lifeboat was contacted. At this point the trawler was 52.33 north and 12.08 west approximately 78 miles from the station. The *John and Margaret Doig* slipped moorings at 12.45 a.m. There was a slight sea. Wind was south-easterly force ½ but visibility was at best 25 metres. The lifeboat reached the trawler at 3.15 a.m. and took the man on board. He was landed at Fenit as this was the nearest point for access to Tralee General Hospital. The lifeboat was back at Valentia at 8.25 a.m.

Ocean Reaper Towed in

On 9 August 2000, Dublin Coastguard notified Mr Foran that the trawler *Ocean Reaper*, with a net on her propeller, was being towed by the fishing vessel *Boy Jason*. The *Boy Jason* had now encountered engine trouble and needed assistance. They were 17.3 miles from the station and north-west of Bray Head. The wind was westerly force five to seven and the sea was rough.

The *John and Margaret Doig* left her moorings at 8.15 a.m. While she was on passage the *Boy Jason* restarted her engine. The lifeboat took over the tow of the *Ocean Reaper* and arrived back at Valentia at 2.05 p.m.

In 2001 the lifeboat launched thirteen times. In the 'Lifeboat in Action' section of *The Lifeboat* magazine the service of the 27 January 2001 was told as follows:

Fire Drama
Coordination between the lifeboat and the Navy was the key to the successful operation to save a blazing Spanish Trawler. Fire had broken out around 3pm on Saturday 27 January (2001) in the accommodation section of the ship, which had twelve people on board.

The *John and Margaret Doig* left Valentia at 3.20pm and headed for the trawler's position fifty-five miles west of Bray Head. Fortunately seas were moderate with good visibility and force five winds but the journey still took two hours. The Irish Naval vessel LE *Aoife* was also in the vicinity and arrived shortly after the lifeboat.

The navy took command of the operation and put a firefighting crew on board the trawler while the lifeboat stood by. After tackling the fire for an hour, the Navy requested that the lifeboat evacuate ten of the Spanish crew members, although the skipper and first mate stayed on board to help the firefighters. The lifeboat then stayed on scene to help the Navy team with the transfer of fire-fighting equipment.

During the transfers, coxswain Seanie Murphy noticed that manoeuvring the lifeboat seemed more difficult than usual so he asked mechanic Leo Houlihan to investigate. He found hydraulic fluid leaking into the steering system due to a broken pipe flange. Thankfully, the problem was not incapacitating but it made Seanie's job far harder than normal as he manoeuvred in 3-4m swells between the two other vessels. It was only thanks to his considerable skill that the lifeboat was able to continue helping. 'It is on occasions like this that team-work really comes into play' said Leo.

The fire fighters had been having difficulty tackling the blaze but at 11.30, after six hours' effort, it was finally brought under control . The lifeboat ferried the 10 crew back to Valentia, arriving at 1.45 a.m. on Sunday morning. During the entire journey, Leo struggled with the steering problem to enable Seanie to get them home.

The *Galaxia* was towed to Valentia. Thanks to the efforts of the Navy and the lifeboat crew, damage was limited to the accommodation and galley areas of the ship and, after a couple of days of repairs, the ship was able to sail back to Spain under its own power. The lifeboat's steering problem was also speedily remedied and she was back on duty soon afterwards.

The Director of Operations of the RNLI sent a collective letter of thanks to Coxswain Seanie Murphy and Crew Members Martin Moriarty, Leo Houlihan (mechanic) Andrew Quigley, Thomas Gilligan, Richard Quigley and Dominic Lyne. Coxswain Seanie Murphy commented 'Nothing Less would be expected of us.'

Cape Verde Islander Lost off Dursey Island

On 22 June 2001, the Valentia and Castletownbere lifeboats were involved in an unsuccessful search. A forty-four-year-old man from the Cape Verde Islands fell overboard from the large tanker *Firth Fisher* 7 miles west of Dursey Island.

Joan of Arc and Eight People Brought in

The *John and Margaret Doig* slipped her moorings at 10.50 a.m. on the 4 September. The *Joan of Arc* had suffered engine failure. She was close to Foher Cliffs in a northerly wind of force five and moderate seas. The lifeboat put a tow rope on board and the angling boat and her crew were towed to safety.

Sick Man Brought Ashore

On 12 October 2001 an emergency call was received from the fishing vessel *Regina Ponti*. She was west of Valentia and 18 miles from the lifeboat station and had an ill crewman on board. The *John and Margaret Doig* set out at 10.30 a.m.

Despite a moderately rough sea and force four south-westerly wind the patient was successfully transferred to the lifeboat. He was landed at 1.15 a.m. into the care of an ambulance crew and taken to hospital. In October 2001 a scroll was presented to Mrs Joan Gallagher. Long-Service Awards were presented to Martin Moriarty and Richard Quigley.

In 2002 Valentia lifeboat launched twenty-five times.

Skellig Dawn assisted twice.
On 26 January 2002 the *Skellig Dawn* suffered machinery failure in gale-force winds and a rough sea. She was north-west of Bray Head and 12 miles from the lifeboat station. The lifeboat *John and Margaret Doig* slipped moorings at 10.55 a.m. She reached the casualty and escorted her to Valentia harbour. Two days later at 8.50 p.m. the lifeboat launched again to the *Skellig Dawn* which was aground at Renard. The lifeboat brought the vessel and her crew to Renard pier where she was secured.

Another *Dawn*

On 2 February 2002 the large fishing vessel *Celestial Dawn* went ashore at the mouth of Dingle harbour. Launching at 7.30 p.m. into force six winds and heavy swells the *John and Margaret Doig* illuminated the area with searchlights and parachute flares. All the crew were safely airlifted in an operation which was successful by virtue of the inter-agency cooperation. The trawler had to be lifted by a crane and removed from the harbour entrance.

A Significant Social Event

At the West County Hotel in Ennis on Easter Monday 2002 the 'Answering the Call' concert was in aid of the RNLI. Phil Coulter and Brian Kennedy were supported by local talent. Amongst the guests were Coxswain Seanie Murphy and Mary from Valentia and Coxswain Ned Dillon and Breeda from Arklow.

In a surprise addition to the programme Phil Coulter presented a painting of Valentia lifeboat to Seanie, and Tess Robinson of the Ennis Branch presented a bouquet of flowers to Mary. This was in recognition of Seanie's twenty years as coxswain at Valentia.

May and August were the busiest months with May having five services and August six. Details appear in the list of services in the appendices.

In 2003 there were seventeen launches. Unusually, though not uniquely, launches to pleasure craft exceeded launches to merchant or fishing vessels. There were eight launches to pleasure craft and five to merchant and fishing vessels.

Help for *Jeanie*

On 17 February 2003, the sail training ship *Jeanie Johnston* experienced adverse conditions. There was a south-easterly gale-force eight wind. She was off the wireless point on Valentia. The local lifeboat was tasked. Launching at 11.15 a.m., the *John and Margaret Doig* saw her safely into the shelter of Valentia harbour and to anchorage at Glanleam. The *Jeanie Johnston* later proceeded to Kells Bay for further shelter.

Eleven Rescued at the Coastguard Patch

On 11 June there was a force eight gale blowing from the south-east. The power boat *Eagle III* suffered machinery failure at the Coastguard Patch off Dolus Head. The *John and Margaret Doig* slipped moorings at 11 a.m. She was quickly on the scene, just over 2 miles from station. A line was secured and the *Eagle III* and her eleven occupants were brought safely to harbour.

A €1 million Rescue

On 14 July 2003, there was a southerly wind force four with a corresponding sea. Some 21 miles west of Bray head and 28 miles from station the large fishing vessel *La Mesange* fouled her prop. At 1 p.m. the *John and Margaret Doig* slipped her moorings. She put a line on board the casualty, valued at €1 million. The vessel and her crew of six were safely landed at Valentia in an operation lasting almost seven hours.

In 2004, the Valentia lifeboat crew spent 255.4 man hours at sea. There were twenty-three launches on service. Twenty were successful. Others coped in two cases and one was a deliberate hoax.

Three Calls in a Week in June

On 6 June 2004, the power boat *Framaria* lost power at 52.05 north 10.29 west over 12 miles from the station. The weather was fine. The *John and Margaret*

Doig slipped moorings at 4.45 p.m. Within two hours she had reached the casualty, secured a tow line and brought the vessel and her four occupants to safety. On the 8 June the lifeboat launched at 8.05 p.m. to the *Ocean Wanderer*, which had suffered machinery failure off Culloo. The wind was southerly force six with a moderate sea. The vessel and her crew of two were brought safely to Valentia.

On 12 June the yacht *Kerry Gannet* fouled her prop one mile west of Dolus head. The lifeboat launched at 11.40 a.m. in fine weather and rendered assistance to the vessel.

Another Three Calls in Another Week in July

On the 5, 8, and 12 July the lifeboat launched. Firstly to the *Star of the Sea* with eight on board one mile north of the Tearaght. She had suffered machinery failure. On 8 July the casualty was the fishing vessel *Phoenix* with two on board. She had machinery failure in the Caherciveen River. On 12 July the *Grainne Maria* with two people on board suffered engine failure north of Bray Head. All the vessels were brought to safe harbour in fine weather.

Nineteen calls occurred in 2005.

Rescue of the Sioux

On 18 April the angling boat *Sioux* suffered machinery failure. She was north of the Wireless Point and 10 miles from the lifeboat station. There was a westerly wind force five and a corresponding sea. The lifeboat set out at 3.25 p.m. and secured a tow line to the casualty. She was towed to Valentia with her eleven occupants on board.

Fire on Spailpin Fanach

On 29 September the trawler *Spailpin Fanach* caught fire west of the Skelligs. Her crew were picked up by the *Arianne*. The lifeboat set out at 4.15 a.m. The four survivors were transferred to the lifeboat and were landed at Valentia at lunchtime. The *Spailpin Fanach* later sank. The events received coverage on national television news bulletins.

On 15 March 2006, the *John and Margaret Doig* engaged on a major voyage. She sailed from Valentia to Aran Islands, Arranmore, Barra Island, Stornaway, Longhope and Buckie Shipyard in north-east Scotland for a refit. The return journey was via the Caledonian Canal. There were nineteen service calls in 2006.

Aground at Dingle

At 4.20 a.m. on 26 March 2006 the relief lifeboat *Volunteer Spirit* slipped moorings. The French trawler *Pors Piron* had grounded at the entrance to Dingle harbour. The lifeboat brought in four of the crew while Dingle Coastguard brought another four to harbour. The master and engineer stayed on board. The *Granuaile*, which was nearby, was put on alert. The local fishing boat *Guiding Star* towed the vessel off the rocks and into Dingle. The Coastguard helicopter inspected the harbour from the air and found no evidence of pollution.

Mine Host to the Rescue

On 6 May 2006, a man sailing a small yacht was seen to be in difficulties off the pier. Vince Kidd, who had recently taken over the Royal Hotel in Valentia, was walking with his son. He saw the situation, returned to his premises and told the people there in the hope that they would call the lifeboat. The lifeboat was presently on the scene but Mr Kidd had entered the water and swam out to the man. He had towed him to safety. The weather conditions were poor and there was an ebb tide. A good job well done.

Two Consecutive Services

On 2 and 3 of August 2006 there were two services. On the 2 the *Marber Therese* fouled her propeller 4 miles west of Bray Head. Launching at 6 p.m., the lifeboat reached the casualty, placed a tow line on board. The vessel and her four crew were landed at Portmagee pier. On 3 August the *Beal Inse* was taking water off Cromwell Point. The lifeboat slipped moorings at 4.30 p.m. and brought the vessel and her crew of two into Valentia. That service lasted thirty minutes.

There were twenty-five launches in 2007.

A Long Run

On the 9 June 2007 the lifeboat set out at 1.10 a.m. The wind was force five with a corresponding sea. The casualty was the yacht *Imarageun*. She was 75 miles west of Valentia. She was reported as dismasted. After thirteen hours at sea the yacht was landed at Valentia. Her crew of two, from London, told of a terrible time at sea and were glad of the rescue.

A Difficult Event

On 13 July the *John and Margaret Doig* brought ashore an injured woman. She had fallen on the Skelligs Rock. She was landed at Renard Point for transfer to Tralee Hospital. While still on board the boat a further call was received. Mr Michael Riordan, a world-famous free climber had been swept of the rocks at the Wireless Point. The lifeboat immediately went to the area. With a flotilla of local boats the area was searched for several days but Mr Riordan was never found.

At the beginning of 2008 the RNLI announced the award of the Gold Badge to Timothy Lyne. The badge was presented in Dublin in May by Coxswain Philip Mc Namara of Donaghadee. There were twenty-three services by Valentia lifeboat in 2008. The most significant services are recorded here.

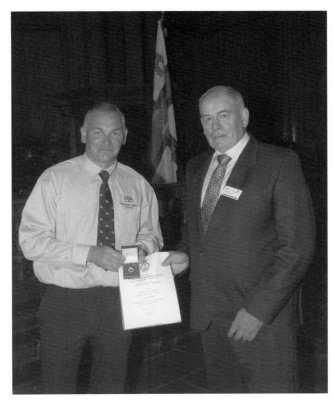

Timothy Lyne is presented with his Gold Badge by Coxswain Philip McNamara of Donaghadee. Photo: courtesy of Margaret Brown.

Wednesday, September 16, 2009
By TED CREEDON

Valentia out in force to honour reluctant heroes

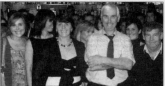

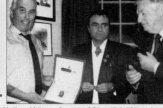

Richard Connolly, right, and Seánie Murphy with his wife Mary and daughters, Shauna, left, Cliona, Bria and Tara at a special function in the Royal Hotel, Knightstown, where both men were honoured for their service to Valentia lifeboat on Friday night. Photos by Ted Creedon

LEFT: Seánie Murphy, left, retiring coxswain of Valentia lifeboat is presented with a commemorative watch by Valentia lifeboat secretary Richard Foran with MC Tommy Gilligan in attendance at a special function in the Royal Hotel, Knightstown, on Friday night.

THE Royal Hotel in Knightstown was packed to capacity on Friday night where the Valentia Island community and guests attended a special function to honour two local men.

Valentia lifeboat coxswain Seánie Murphy and second coxswain Richard Connolly who, between them, have served the local RNLI for more than 70 years have just retired.

Tributes and presentations were made to both men by representatives of the RNLI, the Irish Coast Guard and the Gárda Síochána.

Wellwishers from Dingle and West Kerry also travelled by boat and car to Valentia for the event.

Secretary of Valentia lifeboat Richard Foran told the gathering how both men had been involved in saving hundreds of lives and property over their time of service.

"Seánie was the cox when the Air India disaster occurred in June 1985. People who were with him said he showed true leadership when the lifeboat went to the scene. On October 26 last year Seánie was ill in bed when a call came in that a man had been washed off the cliffs at Culloo. Seánie got out of his bed and took the lifeboat to the location and, in very dangerous conditions, got the boat close enough to rescue the man from the sea. That man was only seconds from death. Seánie showed remarkable skill and dedication and I believe he must go down in history as one of the most remarkable coxswains in the RNLI," he said.

Valentia lifeboat went out more than 120 miles to the scene of the Air India disaster which was beyond the range of its fuel capacity.

The vessel had to be refuelled by naval vessels for its return journey but the rescue exercise showed the dedication and commitment of Seánie Murphy to his post, the gathering was told.

"Richard Connolly spent 41 years with the service. Someone once said that if you put half a dozen eggs down the side of a pier Richard wouldn't crush them when bringing a boat alongside!" Mr Foran said.

RNLI inspector Owen Medland also paid tribute to the men and invited Jeff Mankertz, from RNLI headquarters in Poole, Dorset, to present both men with long service certificates.

A similar certificate for 30 years service was presented to the lifeboat's former mechanic Joe Houlihan on the night.

The Coast Guard rescue helicopter service was represented by Chief Crewman Eamon Ó Briain who made a presentation to Seánie Murphy.

A letter was of congratulations and best wishes on Seánie's retirement from Gárda Superintendent Michael O'Donovan was read out by gárda Tom O'Connell.

The Achill Island lifeboat mechanic Stephen McNulty presented Seánie with a piece of inscribed Achill pottery.

Tony Kehoe from the Rosslare lifeboat also made a presentation to Seánie.

"When I was working fulltime with the lifeboat I spent some time here on the island and stayed in Seánie's mother's house. Best digs in Ireland!" he declared to applause.

Mike McDonnell of Fenit lifeboat had more words of praise for Seánie. John Falvey of the Valentia Coast Guard Station told the audience of Seánie's days as a footballer.

"When I was in goal Seánie played in front of me as full back. He didn't have great speed but he had a great pair of hands. A lot of full forwards went home very sore after playing against him" he said to cheers.

When Seánie was asked to speak he didn't talk about his time with the lifeboat.

Instead, he thanked his family for all their support and he wished the lifeboat crew every success in the future under their new coxswain Richard Quigley.

Saved Boat and Rescued Four Lives

The yacht *Silver Dipper* was north-west of the Blaskets on 27 March 2008. The wind was south-easterly and at near gale force. There was a 4 metre swell and very rough seas. Recognising that they were in difficulties they called for assistance. The lifeboat *John and Margaret Doig* slipped moorings at 5.45 p.m. Fifty minutes after launching she reached the casualty. With great difficulty a tow was established. In view of the difficult conditions, the coxswain decided to pass the casualty drogue to the yacht. This was lost due to the crew being inexperienced. After a tow lasting three and a half hours the casualty and her crew of four was brought safely into Valentia harbour.

Landing the *Flying Horse*

The *Flying Horse* was plying between Ballinskelligs and the Skelligs Rocks on 19 May 2008. She had twelve persons on board. There was a strong south-easterly breeze and a moderate sea but visibility was good. The vessel developed a fuel problem and requested assistance. The lifeboat *John and Margaret Doig* arrived alongside the casualty at 5.05 p.m. just twenty-five minutes after launching. A tow line was passed across and the boat and twelve people were landed at Portmagee pier thirty minutes later.

On 16 August 2008, there was a strong westerly breeze blowing up Dingle Bay. One mile west of Inch Beach a fisherman in his 3 metre boat was seen to be in difficulty. The lifeboat *John and Margaret Doig* was launched to his assistance.

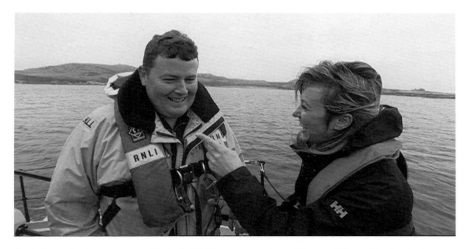

Fresh From the Sea presenter Clodagh Mc Kenna interviews Valentia lifeboat Mechanic Leo Houlihan for a programme for RTE 1 on 30 June 2009. Photo: (C) Inproduction Ltd.

At 4.40 p.m. the lifeboat found the vessel at anchor and passed a line across. The fisherman was advised to cut the anchor cable. The vessel was brought alongside the lifeboat and the fisherman was taken on board. His boat was winched onto the aft deck of the lifeboat and the boat and fisherman were landed in Dingle at tea time.

Another Culloo Victim

On 30 September, in a full gale with rough seas and a heavy swell the *John and Margaret Doig* was launched to a person in the water off Culloo. The lifeboat reached the scene at 4 p.m. The person was taken on board the lifeboat. He failed to respond to medical aid. At Renard pier the local G.P. came on board the lifeboat and the man was pronounced dead.

Man Rescued

A rescue on 26 October 2008 was tricky in its origin, brilliant in its execution and happy in the outcome. Valentia Coastguard Radio was informed of a person in the water. The location was as vague as 'Off Valentia' and in the 'Caherciveen River'. By prudent questioning married to local knowledge it was established that the person was in fact off Culloo. The *John and Margaret Doig* launched into a force seven onshore wind. There were 4 metre swells. Arriving at the cauldron that at that time was Culloo, Coxswain Seanie Murphy with consummate sea-

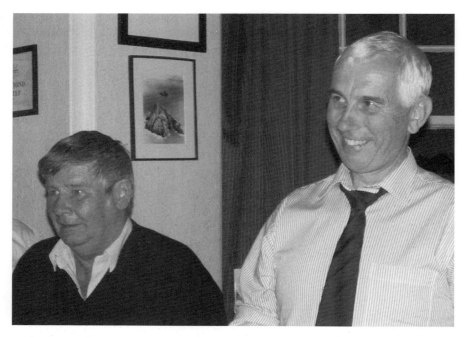

Richard Connolly (second coxswain) and Seanie Murphy (coxswain) on the occasion of their retirement party on 11 September 2009. Photo: Dick Robinson.

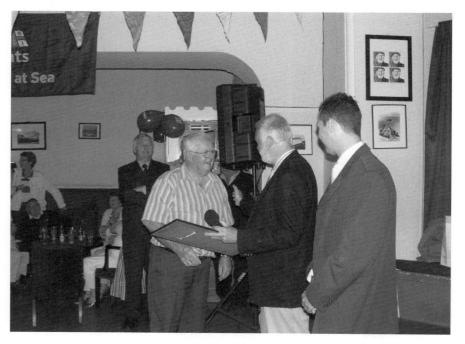

Joe Houlihan receives an award for ten years as DLA. The present Deputy Launching Authorities at Valentia are Timothy Lyne and Nealie Lyne. Photo: Dick Robinson.

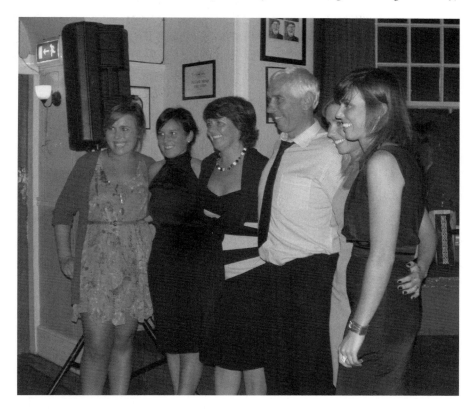

A justifiably proud family. Photo: Dick Robinson.

manship brought the lifeboat within 15 metres of the shore. The casualty was taken on board the lifeboat thereby saving his life. He was landed at Renard pier. Recovering a person from the water in a Severn class lifeboat is not an easy operation. Doing so in the position and in the conditions that obtained on the 26 October 2008 was an outstanding rescue by any standard. It would rate as yet another outstanding rescue in Seanie Murphy's career as coxswain and another tribute to the competence and bravery of his crew.

In August 2009, Seanie Murphy retired after an illustrious career as coxswain. He had held the position since 1 January 1982. From then until the end of 1988 figures indicate 483 launches and 153 lives saved; a proud record indeed.

Also justifiably proud was retiring Second Coxswain Richard Connolly. Having joined the crew in 1968, Richard became second coxswain in 1983. During his service on the lifeboat 273 lives were saved.

Richard Quigley succeeded Seanie as coxswain. Conn O'Shea took over as second coxswain'. In 2009 Valentia lifeboat launched fourteen times and rescued twenty-nine people.

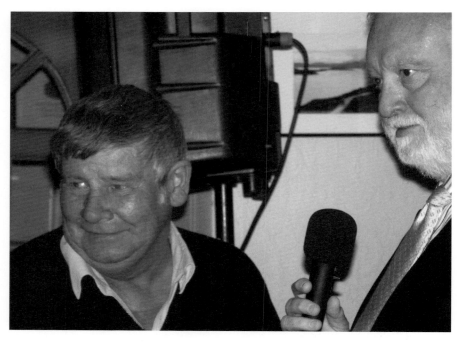

Richard Connolly with Jeff Mankertz. Photo: Dick Robinson.

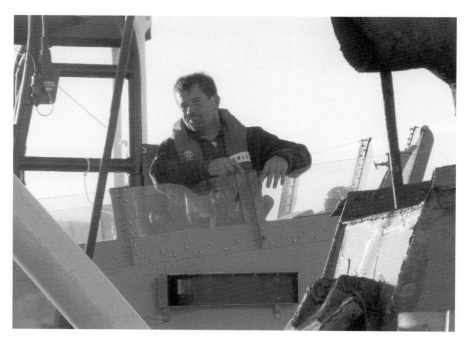

Coxswain Richard Quigley. Photo: Dick Robinson.

EPILOGUE

Ca bhfuil an fear nar phreab a chroí le miain fileadh ar ais mar mhair a sinsear riamh.

There is always a sense of joy and a sense of place for me when I return to this hallowed island of Valentia. The focus never changes. There is the first glimpse of Geokaun Mountain, then the lighthouse, the radio station and the lifeboat moorings and is the boat there.

I saw the first boat come up the harbour in 1946 and watched the arrival of each boat that followed. My early years were spent hanging around the old store at the back of the Watch House. The heroes of my youth and all my years are detailed on the list of crew members.

There is nothing to compare with the adrenaline rush of a call out. In my day the crashing maroons – the race to the boathouse – slipping the moorings – and taking the first sea at the lighthouse.

A study of much RNLI material over some fifty plus years has done nothing to change that. All the books and charts and scrapbooks and videos and DVDs come back to the same basic fact about lifeboat crew: We Save Lives. In Valentia we do it from the most westerly harbour in Europe and in some of the most horrendous seas.

I have tried to the best of my ability to put on record the story of Valentia lifeboat and of the people involved with it. An ever-increasing number of lives saved goes yearly on the record. That no crew person has ever been lost is also on the record and that is a statistic that, please God, will never change. I pray success to Valentia lifeboat crew in all their ventures and adventures.

Now, in the autumn years, I am sure that there are young lads and lassies hanging around the lifeboat station. In fact I know there are, as there are at every lifeboat station for that is what has kept the great service going since 1824.

I hope that amongst that number some one will take photographs and write down the names of people and record the events. I hope too and give my blessing to them to pick up this book, long after I have gone to my reward and say, 'I must bring the Valentia Lifeboat History Up to Date.'

To all who have been involved with Valentia lifeboat in any capacity this book is to say 'I salute you'.

Dick Robinson, 2011

APPENDIX 1

First Twenty-Five Subscribers to Valentia Lifeboat

1. Trinity College, Dublin, £20 and an annual subscription of £3 3s
2. Knight of Kerry, Glanleam, £10 and an annual subscription of £1 1s
3. Lady Molyneaux, £2
4. Marquis of Landsdowne. Bowood Wiltshire, £10 and an annual subscription of £3 3s
5. Daniel O'Connell DL, Derrynane, £5 and an annual subscription of £1 1s
6. James Butler JP, Waterville, £5 and an annual subscription of £1 1s
7. John Fitzgerald JP, Caneagh, £1 and an annual subscription of 10s
8. Captain Needhan, Trinity College, £1 and an annual subscription of 10s 6d
9. Colonel Holden, Dromquinna, an annual subscription of £1 1s
10. Revd John Healy PP, Caherciveen, £1
11. Captain Hartley, Reencurra an annual subscription of £1
12. Dr. Barter, St Anne's, Blarney, £1
13. James Kearney White, Inspecting Chief Office of Coastguard at Caherciveen, £2 and an annual subscription of £1 1s
14. Mr John O'Leary, Victoria Hotel, Killarney, £1
15. Miss Butler of Waterville, £1
16. Dr Barry, JP, Caherciveen, £1
17. Revd John Moore, Caherciveen, £1
18. J. Morragh Bernard DL, High Sheriff, £5 and an annual subscription of £1
19. Richard Mahony DL, Dromore Castl, £3 and an annual subscription of £1 1s
20. Revd. John Fitzgerald Day, Beaufort, £1
21. J. Townsend Trench, Lansdowne Lodge, £2

22. John Leahy JP QC, South Hill, £3 and an annual subscription of £1 1s
23. Capt Harnden of Portmagee, Lobster Fishery, £7
24. Edward B. Hartopp, Melton Mowbray, £5 and an annual subscription of £1
    1s
25. Gerard Connolly, Collector of Customs, 10s

APPENDIX 2

The Beaufort Scale

Force on scale	Nautical MPH	Description	Wave height	Deep sea conditions
0	0 – 1	Calm	–	Flat calm
1	1 – 3	Light airs	¼ (feet)	Small wavelets
2	4 – 6	Light breeze	½	As above with glossy crests
3	7 – 10	Light breeze	2	Large wavelets crests begin to break
4	11 – 16	Moderate breeze	3½	Moderate waves becoming large. Crests break
5	17 – 21	Fresh breeze	6	Moderate waves longer. Crests break
6	22 – 27	Strong breeze	9½	Large waves. Crests break frequently
7	28 – 33	Strong wind	13½	Large waves. Streaky foam
8	34 – 40	Full gale	18	High longer waves, crests from spindrift
9	41 – 47	Strong gale	23	High waves, streaks of foam. Crests roll over
10	48 – 55	Storm	29	Very high seas. Surface white with foam over hanging crests
11	56 – 65	Violent storm	37	Exceptionally high sea, completely covered with foam
12	Above 65	Hurricane		Air full of spray, visibility seriously affected

These are deep sea criteria. Huge waves smashing off cliffs will cause a backwash making coastal waters much more dangerous.

APPENDIX 3

Salvage Claim by Valentia Lifeboat Crew on MV *Ora Et Labora*

Mention the word 'salvage' in maritime environs and you make murder, rape, aggravated assault and burglary pale into insignificance. Immediately you bring to the surface the 'quayside lawyers' speaking with total authority on the Rules of Salvage. Many of these 'experts' have boats which they fear may be the subject of a salvage claim. Many of the boats are such, that were they animals, the only charitable thing to do with them would be to put them down. Everybody has firm opinions of what salvage is not; such terms as legalised piracy etc. have been bandied about for years.

Salvage is a proportion of the value of a ship or cargo paid by insurers or owners to those by whose means they have been saved when in danger, based on prevailing conditions, the labour and danger to the salvor and the salvee. A crew can not claim salvage for saving their own vessel, neither can pilots or passengers or crews of tugs on ordinary duties make a claim. Salvage is not payable when life only is saved.

The RNLI as a body never claims salvage. The crews, as individuals, retain their legal rights to do so. In practice they seldom do. Between 1970 and 1985, Valentia lifeboat crew made one salvage claim and were awarded £1,500 in the

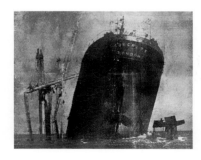

The *Corcrest* sinking. Photo: courtesy of John Steer.

Supreme Court. In the same time the value of property saved by the lifeboat was £2,439,000. The salvage amounted to 0.0615 per cent of the total figure, not an enormous percentage by any standards! This was certainly one of the last if indeed not the last salvage claim lodged by any lifeboat crew.

The basic grounds for making claims are set out in the various Merchant Shipping Acts. Cases stated in the Superior Court in Ireland and Britain are invariably the basis for determination of such claims. The Valentia Salvage Claim 'went the distance' legally, winding up in the Supreme Court, and is reported in the 'Irish Reports' for 1981. The case becomes a precedent for future cases and is worth reproducing for that reason, and to scotch the infantile idea that there is an automatic Rule of Thumb formula for salvage. The case is entitled 'Dermot Walsh, Desmond Lavelle, James Murphy, Patrick Curtin and Aiden Walsh, Plaintiffs -V- An Bord Iascaigh Mhara Defendants, (SC No. 88 of 1977) Admiralty – Salvage – Payment – Assessment – Trawler drifting towards rocks – Trawler towed clear by shore lifeboat – Claim by crew of lifeboat – Fair remuneration'.

On 3 July 1974 the engine of a trawler failed off the coast of Kerry. She began to drift towards rocks offshore in a moderate sea, driven by westerly force six wind. Her distress signal was received and transmitted to Valentia lifeboat, which was launched by 9 p.m. and reached the trawler at 11 p.m. when she was about 200 yards from the rocks. The crew of the lifeboat, the plaintiffs, passed a towline to the trawler and she was towed to safety in port by the lifeboat and her crew. The plaintiffs claimed in the High Court for a salvage award against the Defendants. The trial judge found that the defendant trawler had been saved from destruction or serious damage by the plaintiffs, that the value of the trawler was £45,000 and that the plaintiffs should be awarded £750 to be shared equally by them. On appeal by the plaintiffs it was up held by The Supreme Court (Griffin, Kenny and Parke JJ) in allowing the appeal on the amount of the award, that:

1. Although the lifeboat launched in order to save life and not salve property the plaintiffs were entitled to a salvage award which would remunerate them fairly for their services. 'The Africa Occidental' (1951) 2 Lloyds Rep. 107 considered.
2. That the Salvage Award should be increased to £1,500.

Cases Mentioned in this Report

1. William Bickford, The (1801) 3 CH Rob. 355
2. London Merchant, The (1837) 3HagAdm. 394
3. City of Chester, The (1884) 9 PD 182
4. Annie/The (1886) 12 PD 50
5. Margerite Molinos, The (1903) P.160
6. Rambler, The-v-The Kotka (1917) 2.1.R. 406

7. Kerlogue, The-v-The Wild Rose (1942) IR 28
8. Corcrest, The (1946) LI.L Rep 78
9. Guernsey Coast, The (1950) 83 LI.L Rep. 483
10. Africa Occidental, The (1951) 2 Lloyds Rep. 107

Appeal from the High Court

On 19 February 1975, the plaintiffs issued a summons claiming from the defendants the sum of £75,000 for salvage services rendered to MV *Ora et Labora*, the property of the defendants, off Ducalla Head, in the County of Kerry on 3 July 1974.

The plaintiffs were the coxswain and crew of the lifeboat *Rowland Watts*, a vessel of 25.69 tons which was stationed at Knightstown on Valentia Island. The plaintiffs' action was tried by the president of the High Court on 29 and 30 March and on 1 April 1977, when the president issued an extempore judgement which was recorded by a stenographer. In his judgement the president found that the plaintiffs had rendered salvage services to MV *Ora Et Labora* which was thereby saved from destruction or serious damage, that the plaintiffs were authorised by the owners of the lifeboat to perform those services, that the plaintiffs were entitled to be paid a salvage award, that the value of MV *Ora Et Labora* was £45,000, that the value of the lifeboat was £79,000 and that the amount of the salvage should be £750 to be shared equally by the plaintiffs.

The plaintiffs appealed to the Supreme Court against the Order of the High Court with respect to the amount of the award. The Appeal was heard on 21 and 22 February 1979. R.P. Barr SC (with him A.G. Murphy) for the Plaintiffs referred to the William Bickford, the London Merchant, the City of Chester, the Annie, the Margerite Molinos, the Rambler-v-the Kotka, the Kerlogue-v-the Wild Rose, the Corcrest, the Guernsey Coast, the Africa Occidental. B.M. McCracken SC (with him D.L. Montgomery) for the defendant, referred to the Rambler-v-the Kotka, the Guernsey Coast and the Africa Occidental.
GRIFFIN, J. 6 April, 1979

The facts are fully covered in the judgement of the learned president of the High Court and so only a brief statement of the facts as found by him, is necessary for the purpose of this judgement. The plaintiffs are the coxswain and crew of the Valentia lifeboat. Early in July 1974, the motor trawler *Ora Et Labora*, with an agreed valuation of £45,000, was purchased in Holland by Mr Richard Riordan with the intention of operating it as a trawler out of Dingle. On the 3 July 1974 whilst it was in the course of being brought from Holland to Dingle (with Mr Riordan as skipper, and four other men on board) the engines of the trawler failed when it was east of the Skelligs and approximately one mile from the Lemon Rock off the Kerry Coast. There was at the time a westerly force six wind into a lee shore. The tide was south, one and a half knots and the sea was classified as moderate.

A distress message from the trawler was picked up by Valentia Radio and was treated by them correctly, as found by the president, as a mayday message. In response to that message, the Valentia lifeboat was launched at 9 p.m. From their experience and their knowledge of the waters in the area, the coxswain and crew of the lifeboat calculated that, due to the effects of the wind and tide, the trawler would be likely to drift towards the cliffs near Ducalla Head and Bolus Head, and would be in grave danger not only from these cliffs but also from submerged rocks some two hundred yards off Ducalla Head. The lifeboat reached the trawler at approximately 11 p.m. by which time the trawler was only 400 yards offshore and two hundred yards from the submerged rocks; it was drifting towards both these dangers. The lifeboatmen passed a line to the trawler and towed it away from the rocks and ultimately, towed it to port in Knightstown where it was secured alongside the pier at approximately 4.15 a.m. next morning. The President has found that there was immediate danger of the loss of the motor trawler, which was valued at £45,000. The plaintiffs claim that they are entitled to salvage, based on a proportion of the value of the salved property. Although in the High Court the defendants contested the right of the plaintiffs to any salvage, on the hearing of this appeal they conceded that the plaintiffs were entitled to some salvage; but the defendants submitted that it should be limited to remuneration for the work which the crew of the lifeboat performed. The question for determination on this appeal is, therefore a net one, i.e. where a lifeboat crew are called out to save life and, in the performance of that duty they save the vessel also, how should the salvage to which the crew are entitled be assessed by the court? Under the regulations of the RNLI where a lifeboat has been launched on lifesaving service, which is the primary purpose of the lifeboat, the coxswain and crew are allowed to engage in salvage services to property, in which event they become liable to pay to the Institute the cost of petrol, oil and other consumable stores expended during the service and the cost of any repair to the lifeboat necessitated by accident or otherwise in the course of the service, and the cost of any repairs to, or replacement of, gear damaged or lost during the service. The Institute does not claim salvage nor does it allow salvage to be claimed on its behalf. Therefore, where a salvage claim arises in respect of salvage to property, it is a personal claim by individual lifeboatmen, and is in respect of personal services rendered by the coxswain and members of the crew of the lifeboat, and there can be no claim in respect of services rendered to the salved vessel by the lifeboat itself. The court has to arrive at such an award as will fairly compensate the cox and crew without injustice to the interests of the salved vessel, and encourage others in like circumstances, in the interests of public policy, to perform like services. That would seem to be the underlying principle upon which all awards of salvage are based. Three cases, in each of which claims by lifeboatmen arose, were opened on the appeal and in the High Court. In support of their contention the Plaintiffs relied on *The Corcrest* in which Lord Merriman, President, awarded a total of approximately 40 per cent of the salved ship's value to the salvors, who included the crew of a shore lifeboat. The crew were awarded more than 25 per cent of the entire sum awarded to all the salvors, and that was a substantial sum.

The defendants relied on the *Guernsey Coast* and the *Africa Occidental* in the *Guernsey Coast* the lifeboat was standing by the ship which had gone ground, for approximately one and a half hours and Pilcher J. took the view that, 'the presence of the lifeboat gave them very considerable comfort and moral support'. He awarded £250 to the lifeboatmen for what they did. In the *Africa Occidental* the crew of the lifeboat stood by the ship and, with their experience and local knowledge, gave advice to the pilot. Although the services rendered were small, the crew were held to have conferred a material benefit on the ship, the cargo and freight, and £200 was awarded to them.

The *Corcrest* is distinguishable from the present case. In that case, the *Corcrest* went around in very bad weather on a sandbank, where she was abandoned as a probable total loss: her crew were taken off by the lifeboat which had been called out. Having rescued her crew, the lifeboat returned to its base and safely landed the master and crew of the *Corcrest*. At high tide the *Corcrest* refloated herself and was driving southward in a gale and on the flood tide; it would almost certainly have been wrecked if no further assistance was obtained. In those circumstances, the lifeboat put out again accompanied by a powerful steam tug. The crew of the lifeboat assisted in saving the vessel from certain destruction. On the second occasion there was no question of saving life and the lifeboat men were involved solely in salvage to property. They were, therefore, in the position of ordinary salvors to property, and as such, were held to be entitled to salvage in the same way as the crews of the other vessels involved.

I entirely agree with the learned president that there is a clear distinction between a case in which a lifeboat makes an entire journey with the sole purpose of salvaging a vessel and a case in which the salvaging took place in the course of a voyage to save lives, as occurred in the case of the *Guernsey Coast* and the *Africa Occidental*. I also agree with him that the salvage in this case should not be calculated upon the basis of a proportion of the value of the ship salved but on the basis of remuneration or reward to the lifeboatmen. Mr McCracken, who appeared on behalf of the defendants, submitted that any award to the lifeboatmen should be quite small, otherwise the prospect of a reasonably substantial award might tempt the crew of a lifeboat to save property rather than life, with the possible consequence that life which might otherwise have been saved might be lost.

In my view this is unrealistic and I do not accept it. The crew of a lifeboat are volunteers and are brave and dedicated men. Whatever the weather conditions and the dangers involved, they are prepared to risk their own lives in endeavours to save others whenever a vessel or lives are alleged to be in danger in the area covered by the lifeboat. It should be remembered that it is almost invariably when there are gale-force winds and high seas that vessels get into difficulties. In the case of Valentia lifeboat this area of the Atlantic must be extensive, as the nearest lifeboat station to the south is Baltimore and the nearest north is at Kilronan on the Aran Islands. It seems to me that it would be unthinkable that monetary considerations should in any way influence such men in their primary purpose of saving life, and I believe they would at all times be likely to act in the best interests of those they are endeavouring to save. If, in the course of doing so, they can also salve property, then they are apparently always prepared to do so. Indeed in this case, as the learned president points out in his judgement, in accordance with the ordinary traditions of the sea it did not occur to the lifeboatmen not to make an attempt at least to save the vessel unless they could only do so at the cost of further endangering the lives of those on board the *Ora Et Labora*.

In my opinion the correct basis on which to assess the salvage award is that laid down in the *Africa Occidental* which was the basis adopted by the learned President in his judgement. In that case Willimer J. (as he then was) who had considerable experience of, and was an acknowledged authority in Admiralty Law, said at P.114 of the report:

> During the course of argument I suggested to Mr Bucknill (who appeared on behalf of the defendants) that if, contrary to his submissions, any salvage award was payable, the test for fixing the amount of it should be such a sum as would fairly remunerate those men for what they did, and as would encourage them, and others, to perform similar services in the future as and when the occasion may require ... it seems to me that if lifeboatmen, at their own risk, go beyond what is strictly required for the performance of their main duty of saving life, what they do can only be regarded as highly meritorious and ought to be remunerated by an award which will encourage them, and others, in the future.

To achieve this, the sum awarded should be reasonably generous. In that case Willimer J. awarded £200 which, though he described it as a modest sum, was reasonably generous in the year 1951. In addition, he pointed out in his judgement, the plaintiffs were able to assist the ship only in a small way. In assessing the salvage to which the Plaintiffs are entitled in all the circumstances of this case, the learned president took the view that he should adopt the pattern which was applied in the *Guernsey Coast* and the *Africa Occidental*s which were decided respectively in 1950 and 1951. The lifeboats in those cases involved ten crew, something which he took to be relevant and which gave two figures of £200 and £250. In bringing these figures up to date, the President had regards to the devaluation of money, the fact that five crew members were involved in this case, and that he was trying to assess an award which would encourage them and others.

He assessed the total salvage at £750 including £4 in respect of fuel. In arriving at the remuneration to the plaintiffs therefore, the president took a line through the two cases in 1950 and 1951 where £200 and £250 respectively were awarded. The learned president would appear to have taken the figure of £250 and used a multiplier of six to allow for inflation since 1950-1951 period; then in view of the fact that ten crew were involved in earlier cases and only five crew were involved in this one, he halved the resulting figure of £1,500 to give a remuneration of £750 which he awarded to the plaintiffs. Even though the services provided in the present case conferred a greater material benefit upon the vessel than in the earlier of the two cases in 1950 and 1951, the method adopted by the President for the ascertainment of the remuneration which the plaintiffs should receive was a reasonable one. It was one with which I would agree, except in the respect of the multiplier used. It is remuneration which has to be ascertained. As earnings, or remuneration for work and services, have outstripped the Consumer Price Index, on which the measure of inflation is based, in my view the appropriate multiplier should be that applicable to earnings.

Strange as it may now appear, the average industrial earnings for men in October 1949 were £5 59s (See Irish Statistical Bulletin of June 1951 at P.87). In September 1977, the corresponding figure was £76 85p (See Irish Statistical Bulletin of June 1978 at P.145) which is 13.75 times the earnings at the end of 1949. The corresponding figure for all such employees (i.e. men and women) in 1949 and 1977 respectively were £4 19s and £63 88p; the latter figure being 15.25 times greater than the former. Increases of a somewhat similar order have occurred in the case of agricultural workers and in service industries. In the year 1949 an agricultural worker was entitled under the Agricultural Wages Act to be paid £3 25s for a fifty-four-hour week.

In my opinion therefore, the appropriate multiplier would be twelve — I believe that, if the figures set out in the relevant issues of the Irish Statistical Bulletin had been brought to the attention of the learned president, he would have used a multiplier of twelve so as to give a remuneration of £1,500. As it is only in respect of the multiplier used that I differ from the president (in all other respects I agree fully with his judgement) it would be inappropriate to send the case back to the High Court. Accordingly I would increase the award of £1,500 and allow the appeal.

KENNY, J.

I have read the judgement of Mr. Justice Griffin and I agree with it.

PARKE, J.

I have had an opportunity to read the judgement of Mr. Justice Griffin and I also agree with it.

Solicitors for the Plaintiffs: Coakley, Moloney & Flynn. Solicitors for the Defendants: Thomas Montgomery & Son. Seeing in full the detail in which all aspects of the case will be considered and the precedent cases examined must convey that being said and led by the 'Quayside Lawyer' is, to say the least, unwise. It also reinforces the legal maxim 'He who conducts his own case has a fool for a client'. 'Nailed to the mast' has become such an everyday expression that many people are unaware that it is in fact referring to the method of serving Admiralty Summonses and other documents. In the case of the *Ora Et Labora* that time-honoured method of service was also envisaged. A Civil Process Server from north Kerry was dispatched to Dingle with his Legal Document, a claw hammer and a stalwart nail. Having located the *Ora et Labora* he proceeded in the maritime tradition by nailing the Bill to the Mast. Unfortunately he failed to take account of the fact that the mast was made of steel. Fortunately his remarks on making the discovery in the above fashion are not recorded. With typical north Kerry resilience he obtained adhesive tape and the document was 'Taped to the Mast' and while legally effective it lacks the poetic ring to make it an everyday cliché.

The RNLI has a rigid policy of not claiming salvage. This was also the policy in the last century. Then however the Institution took a portion of the salvage money equal to the shares of two crewmen to cover the risk of damage to the lifeboat. A bitter row over salvage broke out at Eastbourne, Sussex in 1884. The previous November the lifeboat had been taken 5 miles overland, launched with great difficulty and eleven survivors were rescued from a barque. The following day the neighbouring Newhaven lifeboat accompanied a tug which towed the barque to harbour. Newhaven crew were involved solely in a salvage operation and could lawfully make claim. Vexed by this turn of events, the Eastbourne men, although paid double the normal service fee by the RNLI, £20 by the donor of the lifeboat, and £70 raised by the people of the town as a tribute, claimed live salvage. Despite warnings from the RNLI, they accepted £150 from the ship's owners. The entire crew was dismissed and a boathouse keeper was appointed. In the event of a shipwreck he was instructed to give the boathouse keys to any group of competent men demanding them.

The *Corcrest* referred to in the case had indeed some RNLI significance, Cromer lifeboat in Norfolk was the lifeboat involved with her. The service took place on 7 March 1946. The lifeboat assisted to save the vessel and rescued 22. This was the last effective launch in command of the lifeboat for the legendary Coxswain Henry Blogg. (Titled as 'The Greatest of the Lifeboatmen', Blogg had been on the crew for over fifty years of which he was coxswain for thirty-eight. During his years of service Cromer lifeboat launched 387 times and saved 873 lives. He held three gold and four silver medals and the George Cross.) The *Corcrest* herself ran aground on the wreck of the *Fort Massac* north-west of the Sunk Light vessel off the Essex Coast on 22 June 1949.

Efforts to salvage her were not successful and her crew of twenty-three, and ten salvage men and ten marine superintendents were rescued by the Walton and Frinton lifeboat.

APPENDIX 4

List of Services Performed by Valentia Lifeboat Including
Statistical Analysis

Services 1946–1969

Date	LB	Casualty	Cause	Assessment
1946				
26/12/1946	690		Distress signals	False alarm
(C and S)				
1947				
12/01/1947	690		Body on Blaskets	Landed at Dingle
23/04/1947	680	(*City of Bradford 1*)	Vessel adrift	Towed to pier
18/09/1947	687	(*BASP*)	Distress flares	False alarm
1948				
17/02/1948	687	FV *Marie*	Overdue	False alarm
10/04/1948	680	FV *Naomh Seaghan*	Overdue	Saved boat/rescued 4
19/06/1948	680	FV *Naomh Fiontan*		Others coped
23/08/1948	680	Yacht *Crimson Rambler* of Lymington		False alarm

1949				
22/03/1949	680	FV *Morning Star* of Caherciveen		Saved boat/rescued 4
29/04/1949	687	(*BASP*) FV *Ocean Star* of Dingle	Overdue	Assistance not required
27/06/1949	687	Small rowing boat	Adrift	Boat escorted/saved 5
14/10/1949	687		Distress flares	False alarm
1950				
23/01/1950	687	FV *San Pedro*	Missing	Search failed
22/02/1950	687	FV *Pride of Ballinskelligs*		Saved boat/rescued 2
24/03/1950	687	Skelligs Lighthouse		Relieved lighthouse
24/03/1950	687	Tearaght Lighthouse		Relief not possible due to weather
26/03/1950	687	Tearaght Lighthouse		Relieved lighthouse
01/08/1950	687	FV *Ocean Star*	Overdue	Escorted vessel to Dingle Lighthouse
16/09/1950	687	Boat from MV *St Bravels* of Newport		Found safe ashore at Glanleam
16/09/1950	687	FV *Amazone* of Finisterre, France		Escorted into Valentia harbour
16/10/1950	687	FV *Jundina* of Vigo		Others coped
1951				
30/01 1951	687	Dredger *Samphire* of Cobh Fenit	Lifeboat reported drifting, mine 4 miles northwest of lighthouse	Fenit lifeboat coped
23/03/1951	717	(AED) American Air Craft		Stood by at station
23/03/1951	717	French trawler *Globemaster*	Reported in distress	False alarm
17/04/1951	717	SS *Fort Enterprise* of London	Injured man	Took out doctor and landed casualty

25/04/1951	717	FV *Naomh Donhaill* of Portmagee		Others coped
05/05/1951	717	FV *Pride of Caherciveen*		Saved boat/rescued 4
10/08/1951	717		Aircraft might have to ditch in Dingle Bay	Stood by (landed safely)
21/08/1951	717		Distress rockets	False alarm
29 & 30/09/1951	717	FV *Maria Natiyidad* Pasajes, Spain	Missing	Searches failed
1952				
04/01/1952	717	Blasket Islands	Cut off for four weeks	Landed food and medical supplies for 28 inhabitants
06/01/1952	717	MV *Plassey* of Limerick		Stood by
02/05/1952	717	FV *Amazone* of Camaret		Stood by
20/06/1952 (*KECF*)	700	Inbound flight from USA		Stood by on board
1953				
12/01/1953	717	*Lydia* of Stettin		False alarm
03/02/1953	717	Skelligs Rock Lighthouse		Relieved lighthouse
09/04/1953	717	FV *Ros Ruadh* of Dublin		Saved boat/rescued 4
06/05/1953	717	FV *Naomh Cait* of Dublin		Others coped
14/05/1953	717	FV *Liberator* of Camaret, France		Saved boat/rescued 9
11/08/1953	717	Swimmer	Missing	Search failed
16/09/1953	717	Punt	Capsized	Recovered punt/rescued 2
12/10/1953	717	FV *Ros Corr* of Dublin		Saved Boat/rescued 6
16/11/1953	717	Skelligs Rock Lighthouse	Injured man	Took out relief keeper and landed casualty

1954				
18 & 19/02/1954	717		Distress rockets	False alarm
20/02/1954	717	Trawler *River Spey* of Milford Haven		Saved boat/rescued 12
12/03/1954	717	FV *Ros Corr* of Dublin		Gave help
04/04/1954	717	Skelligs Rock Lighthouse	Injured man	Landed casualty
20/04/1954	717	FV *Island Rover* of Tralee		Saved boat/rescued 4
08/05/1954	717	Trawler *Brecon Castle* of Swansea	Injured man	Took out nurse and landed casualty
01/06/1954	717	FV *Ros Corr* of Dublin		Gave help
12/06/1954	700	(*KECF*) FV *Naomh Fiontan* of Portmagee		Gave help
17/06/1954	700	FV *Nono* of Caramet, France		Gave help
02/11/1954	717	FV *Casthelios* of Vigo, Spain		Gave help
26/11/1954	717	FV *Ros Airgead* of Dublin		Gave help
01/12/1954	717	Skellig Rock Lighthouse	Ill man	Landed casualty
10/12/1954	717	Inistearaght Lighthouse	Ill man	Landed casualty
19/12/1954	717	Inistearaght Lighthouse	Ill man	Landed casualty
1955				
06/06/1955	717	Yacht MAB		Saved boat/rescued 2
08/06/1955	717	FV *Ros Airgead* of Dublin		Gave help
17/06/1955	717	Fishing Boat *Scadan*		Gave help
06/08/1955	717	FV *Naomh Cionnec* of Dublin		Saved boat/rescued 11
17/11/1955	717	FV *Styvel* of Concarneau, France		Rescued 10

1956				
03 & 04/05/1956	717	FV *Notre Dame des Victores* of Lorient		Fenit lifeboat also involved in search, third search failed fourth located wreckage
03/06/1956	717	*Guillaume Anna Marie* of France		With aid of another trawler vessel 12 crew landed at Valentia
06/06/1956	717	FV *Carrigdoun* of Dublin		Assisted to rescue 1
22/07/1956 (*William and Harriott*)	718	Tanker *Dona Myrto* of Panama	Ill man	Landed casualty
21 & 22/08/1956	717		Keeper missing off Skelligs Rock Lighthouse	Search failed
24/08/1956	717		Further search at request of Commissioners of Irish Lights	Search failed
05&06 /10/1956	717	Flares off the Bull Rock Lighthouse		Search failed
17/18 /10/1956	717	Trawler *Mardemingo B* of San Sabastian		Search failed
17 & 18/11/1956	717		Flares reported	False alarm
1957				
06/03/1957	717	MFV *Acasia* of Dublin		Saved boat/rescued 6
28/05/1957	717	Tanker *Harvella* of London	Ill man	Took out doctor and nurse and landed casualty
05/06/1957	717	FV *Naomh Cait* of Dublin		Saved boat/rescued 5
12/06/1957	717		Stood by for test helicopter landing	Test landing abandoned at Skelligs Rock Lighthouse due to dense fog
04/08/1957	717	Row boat		Others coped

1958				
09/04/1958 (*William and Harriott*)	718	FV *Ros Caoin* of Dublin		Saved boat/rescued 6
04/06/1958 (*Rowland Watts*)	938	FV *Maria* of Waterford		Stood by and gave help
18/06/1958	938	FV *Maria* of Waterford		Saved boat/rescued 3
25/06/1958	938	Trawler *Naomh Cait* of Dublin		Saved boat/rescued 5
10/08/1958	938	MV *Dun Aengus* of Dublin		Gave help
09/12/1958	938	Motor Boat *Spray of Tralee*		Saved boat/rescued 2
1959				
26/01/1959	938	FV *Virgin De La Guia* of Spain		Escorted vessel
07/02/1959	938	FV *Marie Brigette* of Concarneau		Landed 2 bodies and wreckage
20/05/1959	938	FV *Lough Loy* of Dublin		Others coped
30/07/1959	938	BOAC Plane		Alert cancelled
14/08/1959	938	FV *Maragita Lopez* of San Sabastian		Vessel towed clear of Beginish Island (Valentia harbour)
20/08/1959	938	TWA Flight		Stood by
19/09/1959	938	Air France Plane	Missing	Stood by
03/10/1959	938	Canoe (Smerwick)		Search failed
16/10/1959	938	Open motor boat		False alarm
17/11/1959	938	FV *Ros Airgead* of Dublin		Saved boat/rescued 6
13/15 11 1959		Lifeboat off moorings due to hurricane		Sheltered at Beginish Island
19/12/1959	938	Aircraft alert Pan American		Stood by
1960				
09/03/1960 (*Peter and Sarah Blake*)	755	FV *Ros Corr* of Dublin		Saved boat/rescued 5

13/04/1960	938	FV *Santa Catalina* of Spain		Alert cancelled
06/08/1960	938	FV *Ros Bui* of Dublin		Saved boat/rescued 6
05/09/1960	938	FV *Ros Ceaoin* of Dublin		Saved boat /rescued 5
09/09/1960	938	Bather		Landed a body
07/11/1960	938	Piper Apache Aircraft		Plane landed safely/ lifeboat recalled
16/12/1960	755	FV *Ros Airgead* of Dublin		Saved boat/rescued 6
19/12/1960	755	FV *Ros Airgead* of Dublin		Saved boat/rescued 6
1961				
26/02/1961	755			Conveyed surgical team to island
15/05/1961	755	FV *Ros Bui* of Dublin		Saved boat/rescued 6
31/05/1961	755	Aircraft		Stood by
01/07/1961	755	Tearaght Lighthouse	Injured man	Landed casualty
06/12/1961	938	FV *Pience Paysanne* of France		Crew came ashore in rafts. Lifeboat recalled
1962				
17/01/1962	938	FV *Abregaron*		Alert cancelled
31/08/1962	755	Yawl with 6 children on board		Escorted vessel
17/10/1962	938	FV *Pride of Ballinskelligs*	Vessel in tow of FV *Ros Airgead*	Escorted vessels into harbour
1963				
7&8/4/1963	938	Small boat	Capsized	Boat taken to Renard Point
15/06/1963 (*Mary Stanford*)	733	Skelligs Rock Lighthouse	Ill man	Landed casualty
19/06/1963	938	Diver		Body recovered by Des Lavelle
1&2/07/1963	938	MV *Venturer*		Vessel arrived in Derrynane. Alert cancelled
30/07/1963	938	Fibreglass dinghy		Landed at Flesk Cove. Alert cancelled

10/08/1963	938	FV *Ros Ailither* of Dublin		Saved boat/rescued 5
03/09/1963	938	Cargo Ship *Holmfield* of Liverpool		Gave help
09&10 /12/1963	938	FV *Mary Immaculate* of Lisnskea. Northern Ireland vessel		Arrived at Kilbaha, Co. Clare. Lifeboat recalled.
21/12/1963	938	Cargo Ship *Wellpark* of Glasgow	Injured man	Took out doctor and nurse and landed a casualty
1964				
12/05/1964	938		Ill woman	Conveyed casualty to Renard Point
21/06/1964	938	FV *Vispon* of La Corruna, Spain in tow of FV *Muella*		Escorted vessels to Bantry
25/08/1964	733		Distress flares	False alarm
13/09/1964	733		Distress flares	Search failed
28/11/1964	938		Shouts for help	Caherciveen River Garda had no word of missing persons. Lifeboat recalled
04/12/1964	938	Cargo Vessel *Waldemar Peter* of Hamburg	Ill man	Took out doctor and landed a body
1965				
24/04/1965	733	Trawler *Revellin* of Cueta, Spain		Saved boat/rescued 14
19/07/1965	733	Punt with outboard motor		Gave help
25/10/1965	938	Skelligs Rock Lighthouse	Injured man	Landed casualty
28/12/1965	938	MV *Maracove*	Injured man	Took out doctor and landed casualty
1966				
02/03/1966	938	Tanker *Esso Canterbury* of London	Injured man	Landed casualty
03/08/1966	733	Bather		Landed a body
29/08/1966	938	Small fishing boat		Escorted vessel

14/09/1966	938		Persons stranded on Blaskets	Landed 1
1967				
22/01/1967	938	Tanker *Irish Holly*		Gave help
28/01/1967	938	Rowing Boat		Saved boat/rescued 2
03/04/1967	938	Diver in Lough Kay		Search failed
05/05/1967	733	FV *Beal Inse* of Dublin		Saved boat/rescued 11
07/06/1967	938	MV *Iron Ore*		Landed an injured man
22/06/1967	938	Motor Boat *Tralee*		Gave help/ rescued 7
30/07/1967	938	MV *Praunheim* of Bremen	Injured man	Landed casualty
17/09/1967	938	Bull Rock Lighthouse		Landed crew member
16/10/1967	938	MV *Ginnheim* of Germany		Took out a doctor
1968				
17/07/1968	755	MV *Lios Dairbre*		Gave help
30/07/1968	755	Inistearaght Lighthouse	Injured man	Landed casualty
22/12/1968	938	FV *Sea Flower*	Missing	Search failed
1969				
23/01/1969	938	MV *Thelka* of Norway		Saved boat/rescued 14
11/06/1969	938	FV *Ros Molt*		Saved boat/rescued 4
22/06/1969	938	MFV *Siveen*		Saved boat/rescued 5
22/06/1969	755	MFV *Siveen*		Gave help
23/06/1969	755	MFV *Eilis* of Dublin		Saved boat/rescued 5
25/06/1969	755	MFV *Kells Bay*		Saved Boat/rescued 4
01/07/1969	755	MFV *Lios Dairbre*		Gave help
13/07/1969	755	Passenger Vessel *Skellig Michael*		Others coped
20/07/1969	755		People stranded on Great Blasket	Rescued 12
09/10/1969			Fire on Blaskets	Man taken off island
23/10/1969		FVG *Granat*		Saved vessel/landed 5

Services 1970–1989

Date	LB	Casualty	Cause	Assessment
1970				
30/01/1970 (*Rowland Watts*)	938		Distress signal	False alarm
20/02/1970	938	MV *Oranmore*		Rescued 10/landed a body
23/05/1970 (*Peter and Sarah Blake*)	755		People stranded on Skelligs	Landed 15
06/06/1970	755	FV *Siveen*		Landed casualty
07/06/1970	755	Two skin divers		Landed 2
18/07/1970	755	MFV *Granat*		Escorted vessel
27/08/1970	755		Vessel overdue	Alert cancelled/no launch
27/08/1970	755		FV overdue	Others coped
28/08/1970	755		Sick man on Inistearaght Lighthouse	Gave help
17/11/1970	755	Spanish vessel *Mero of Vigo*	On fire	Others coped
12/12/1970	938	Aircraft		False alarm
1971				
01/05/1971	938	Vessel *One More Time*	Overdue	Others coped
09/07/1971	938		Distress signal	Search failed
16/07/1971	938		Vessel overdue	Others coped
01/08/1971	938	Rowing boat		Saved boat
04/08/1971	938	FV *Gan Eagle* of Cork		Saved boat/rescued 2
24/08/1971	938	Yacht *True Light* in tow of MFV *Eilis*		Landed casualty
31/08/1971	938	Tug *Gnat* and Barge		Escorted casualty
25/09/1971	755	MFV *St Colette* of Dublin		Saved boat/rescued 5
01/10/1971	755	Ship *George X* of Greece		Stood by vessel
09/10/1971	755		Distress signal	Search failed
07/11/1971	938		Vessel overdue	Search failed
09/11/1971	938	Fishing vessel	Missing	Search failed
17/11/1971	938		Distress signal	Hoax probably

1972				
31/01/1972	938		Body in the sea	Search failed
21/02/1972	938	MFV *Orion* of Skibbereen		Saved boat/rescued 7
24/02/1972	938	MFV *Ard Fionbarr* of Dublin		Saved boat/rescued 5
24/03/1972	938	Small fishing boat		Saved boat/rescued 1
05/04/1972	938	Ship *Eric Weinerp* of Germany		Stood by
16/06/1972	938	MFV *Dairbhre*		Saved boat/rescued 1
31/07/1972	938	Small fishing vessel	Fouled propeller	Others coped
15/08/1972	938		Distress signal	False alarm
24/08/1972	938	FV *Eilis*	Overdue	Others coped
07/10/1972	938	Skelligs Rock Lighthouse		Took out relief keeper and landed an injured man
09/11/1972	938	Spanish trawlers *Monte Izankun* and *Costa de Isloda*		Gave help
15/11/1972	938	MFV *Donamaur*	Fouled propeller	Landed casualty
1973				
02/02/1973	938		Two people stranded on Beginish Island	Rescued 2
13/04/1973	938	Skelligs Rock Lighthouse	Ill man	Landed casualty
23/04/1973	938	Unnamed vessel in trouble		Others coped
17/05/1973	938	Spanish Trawler *Eilris*	Ill man	Escorted helicopter
07/07/1973	938	Fishing vessel *Puerta Areas* of Spain	Ill man	Stood by
12/08/1973	938		Distress signals	Search failed
24/08/1973	938	Greek cargo ship (name unknown)	Ill man	Landed casualty
18/10/1973	938	Spanish FV *Costallana*	Ill man	Gave help

16/11/1973	938	French Factory Ship *Victor Pleven*	Ill man	Escorted helicopter
1974				
07/02/1974	938	Skellig Rock Lighthouse		Gave help
12/04/1974	938	Skellig Rock Lighthouse		Gave help
07/05/1974	938		Vessel capsized	False alarm
03/07/1974	938	MFV *Ora Et Labora*		Saved boat/rescued 5
16/07/1974	938	Surf board		Others coped
04/08/1974	938	Rowing boat	Over due	Others coped
15/08/1974 (*City of Edinburgh*)	802		Ill man	Others coped
21/08/1974	802	Spanish trawler	Ill man	Escorted helicopter
31/08/1974	802	MFV *Don Mavir*		Landed casualty
30/09/1974	802		Vessel capsized	Others coped.
02/11/1973 (*John Gallantly Hyndham*)	923	Spanish FV *Oneagra*	Injured man	Others coped
1975				
02/02/1975	923	MFV *Spailpin Fanach*		Escorted vessel
22/03/1975	923	MFV *Granat*		Saved boat/rescued 5
30/05/1975	923	MFV *Rosebud*		Landed casualty
16/06/1975	923	MFV *Granat*		Landed casualty
10/08/1975	923	MFV *Valkyrie*		Others coped
13/10/1975	923	MFV *Granat*		Landed casualty
15/12/1975	923	MFV *Granat*		Saved boat/rescued 5
1976				
29/02/1976	938	MFV *Granat*		Others coped
09/03/1976	938	MFV *Ard Fionbhar*		Saved vessel
08/05/1976	938	Bull Rock Lighthouse	Ill man	Landed casualty
10/05/1976	388		Persons stranded on Inishvickillane	Landed 2
02/07/1976	938	MFV *Granat* of Dublin		Landed casualty
25/07/1976	938	MFV *Mary Sue* of Dublin		Landed casualty

08/08/1976	938		Distress signals	Hoax probably
14/08/1976	938	Man overboard from small boat		Search failed
30/08/1976 (*Euphoysne Kendal*)	912		Large fishing vessel	Casualty reached Ballydavid
11/12/1976	938	MFV *Spailpin Fanach*	Ill man	Gave help
11/12/1976	938	MFV *St Colette*	Man overboard	Search failed
1977				
25/04/1977	938	Spanish trawler	Ill man	Escorted vessel
23/06/1977	938	MFV *Granat* of Dublin		Landed casualty
23/08/1977	938	Sailing yacht of Howth		Others coped
26/09/1977	938	MFV *Beal Inse* of Dublin		Landed casualty
14/10/1977	938	Ships lifeboat capsized		Saved vessel
08/12/1977	938	Persons stranded on Inisvickillane		Gave help
1978				
07/02/1978	938	MFV *Granat* of Dublin		Others coped
24/04/1978 (*Joseph HiramChadwick*)	898		Distress signals	False alarm
24/06/1978	898		Vessel overdue	Search failed
12/07/1978	898	Spanish trawler	Ill man	Landed casualty
16/08/1978	898		Manual craft leaking	Search failed
17/08/1978	898		Persons missing	Search failed
23/08/1978	898	Rig supply vessel		False
03/10/1978	898		Person drowning	Search failed
1979				
08/02/1979	898	MFV *Ora et Labora*		Search failed
22/02/1979	938	French fishing vessel		Others coped
10/05/1979	938	Two French trawlers		Others coped

20/06/1979	938	MFV *Rosebud* of Dublin		Landed casualty
10/07/1979	938	MFV *Jackdaw* of Dublin		Landed casualty
16/07/1979	938	MFV *Beal Inse* of Dublin		Landed casualty
29/08/1979	938	MFV *Sea Quest*		Others coped
04/09/1979	938	Sailing dinghy *Dingaleen*		Others coped
07/09/1979	938	MFV *Orion* of Dublin		Escorted vessel
09/09/1979	938	MFV *Lady Jane* of Dublin		Landed 2
1980				
04/04/1980	938	Yacht *Machrista*		Saved boat/rescued 5
16/06/1980	938	MFV *Christian Island* of Cork		Landed casualty
04/07/1980	938	MFV *Welcome Home* of Tralee		Saved boat/rescued 3
16/09/1980	938	Canoe	Overdue	False alarm
02/10/1980	938	Small powered vessel		False alarm
02/10/1980	938	Spanish trawler		Escorted vessel
05/11/1980	938	MFV *Dancing Wave* of Cork		Landed casualty
18/12/1980	938	Tanker *Authenticity* of London		Stood by vessel
30/12/1980	938		Person missing	Search failed
31/12/1980	938		Person missing	Search failed
1981				
13/06/1981	912	MFV *Interceptor* of Cork		Saved boat/rescued 5
24/07/1981	912	MFV *Ocean Wanderer* of Cork		Landed casualty
25/07/1981	912	MFV *Dalmatian Guernsey* of Spain		Saved boat/rescued 9
1982				
28/01/1982	938	MFV *Rob Sisa* of Spain	Ill man	Landed casualty
04/03/1982	938	MFV *Spailpin Fanach*		Landed casualty

11/03/1982	938	MV *Ranga* of Spain		Others coped
13/06/1982	938	Rowing boat	Capsized	Search failed
16/06/1982	938	MFV *Emma Jane*		Saved boat/rescued 2
28/06/1982	938	MFV *Robriza* of Falmouth		Landed casualty
26/07/1982	938	MFV *Ocean Wanderer* of Cork		Landed casualty
03/08/1982	938	Motor cruiser *Wanderer* of Dublin		Landed casualty
22/08/1982	938	MFV *Shooting Star* of Tralee		Saved boat/rescued 2
26/08/1982	938		Persons drowning	Others coped
08/09/1982	938	MFV *Welcome Home* of Tralee		Landed casualty
07/10/1982	938	MFV *Welcome Home* of Tralee		Others coped
11/10/1982 (Last service launch at Valentia)	938	MFV *Ard Beara*	Man overboard from	Others coped
1983				
09/04/1983 (*Margaret Frances Love*)	1082	MFV *Kalernec* of France		Landed casualty
13/06/1983	1082		Skin diver	Others coped
10/09/1983	1082		Distress flares	False alarm
28/09/1983	1082	MFV *Dancing Wave* of Cork		Landed casualty/ rescued 3
06/10/1983	1082	Cargo Vessel *Penelope Everard*		Others coped
17/11/1983	1082	*An Tam Realtoir* of Dublin		Others coped
1984				
11/02/1984	1082		Vessel capsized	False alarm
03/05/1984	1082	MFV *Marita Anne* of Tralee		Saved boat/rescued 3
18/05/1984	1082	MFV *Anticomus* of France		Took out doctor/ landed sick man
29/06/1984	1082	Large French MFV		Escorted vessel

30/06/1984	1082	MFV *St Anthony*		Saved boat/rescued 3
10/07/1984	1082	Sail board		Others coped
10/07/1984	1082	Small FV in tow of MFV *Carol Ann*		Stood by
14/07/1984	1082	MFV *Ardent II*		Saved boat/rescued 6
19/07/1984	1082	Canoe	Vessel capsized	False alarm
25/07/1984	1082	MFV *Naomh Breannan*		Landed casualty
06/08/1984	1082		Distress signal	False alarm
25/08/1984	1082	Skelligs Rock Lighthouse	Ill man	Took out doctor/ landed casualty
26/08/1984	1082	Five persons stranded on Scarriff Island		Gave help
08/09/1984 (*Hyman Winstone*)	1067	Spanish trawler *Jose Delores*	Man overboard	Search failed
17/09/1984	1067	MFV *Interceptor* of Cork		Saved boat/rescued 2
21/09/1984	1067	MFV *Salandina* of Spain		Gave help
13/10/1984	1067		Person missing	Search failed
14/10/1984	1067		Person missing	Search failed
17/12/1984	1082		Distress signal	False alarm
1985				
12/01/1985	1082	MFV *Fortune Hunter*		Saved boat/rescued 3
14/03/1985	1082	Rowing boat	Man overboard	Others coped
19/03/1985	1082	MFV *Haugagut* of Norway	Ill man	Stood by
18/04/1985	1082		Distress signal	False alarm
24/04/1985	1082	MFV *Ronan Padraigh* of Tralee	Ill man	Landed casualty
26/04/1985	1082	MFV *Santa Susana* of Penzance	Ill man	Patient airlifted by RAF
28/04/1985	1082	Small fishing boat	Overdue	Saved boat
23/06/1985	1082	Air India flight 182	Crashed in Atlantic	Landed 5 bodies
04/08/1985	1082		Distress signal	False alarm
10/08/1985	1082		Distress signal	False alarm

21/08/1985	1082	Sail board in adverse conditions		Others coped
29/09/1985	1082	Yacht *Taurima* of Dublin		Crew rescued by Baltimore lifeboat
10/11/1985	1082		Girl trapped on cliff face	Gave help
14/12/1985	1082		Helicopter in trouble	Stood by
1986				
27/03/1986	1082	MFV *Agnes Oilbhear*		Saved boat/rescued 1
28/03/1986	1082	Cargo ship *Mull of Georgetown*		Stood by
02/05/1986	1082		Distress signal	Search failed
27/05/1986	1082	Yacht *Patrick Sarsfield* of Limerick		Saved boat/rescued 5
12/06/1986	1082	Yacht *Cobolt Blue*		Landed casualty
02/07/1986	1082	MFV *Eilis*		Landed casualty
11/07/1986	1082	MFV *Patos Wish*		Landed casualty
16/07/1986	1082	Sailboard		Others coped
19/07/1986	1082	Powerboat *Joyina* of Limerick		Others coped
26/07/1986	1082	MFV *Ard Fionbarr*		Saved boat/rescued 5
14/08/1986	1082	MFV *Ocean Mist*		Others coped
25/08/1986	1082	Yacht *Sigmet*		Saved boat/rescued 2
07/09/1986	1082	Small boat	Overdue	False alarm
26/09/1986	1082	Yacht *Cumbrae*		Landed casualty
30/09/1986	1082	MV *Holger* of Germany		Gave help
16/11/1986	1082	MV *Humbergate*		Stood by
18/11/1986	1082	Tanker *Capo Emma* of Italy		Alert cancelled
19/11/1986	1082	MFV *Ailsa Grace*		Saved boat/rescued 1
20/11/1986	1082	MV *Deresa*		Others coped
16/12/1986	1082	MV *Fait Sultare*		Escorted vessel

1987				
14/03/1987	1082	MV *Kilkeel Lass*		Escorted vessel
18/04/1987	1082	Power boat		Others coped
26/04/1987	1082	FV *Tercero Riocil*	Man overboard	Recovered body
05/05/1987	1082	FV *San Pablo* of Spain	Injured man	Landed casualty
19/05/1987	1082	FV *Ronan Padraig*	Injured man	Landed casualty
12/06/1987	1108	(Margaret Russell Fraser) MV *Dawn Crest*		Landed casualty
27/06/1987	1108		Vessel overdue	False alarm
03/07/1987	1108	MFV *Boston Whirlwind*	Injured man	Landed casualty
18/07/1987 (Ex-RNLB *Mary Stanford*)	1108			Saved boat/rescued 3
23/07/1987	1108		Distress signal	False alarm
01/08/1987	1108	Yacht *Midnight Owl*		Landed casualty
02/08/1987	1108	Fishing vessel	Ill man	Landed casualty
12/08/1987	1108		Distress signals	False alarm
26/08/1987	1108		Vessel stranded	Others coped
13/09/1987	1108		Distress signals	Search failed
14/09/1987	1108	Skin diver	Missing	False alarm
08/11/1987	1082	Fishing vessel	Swamped	Others coped
92/12/1987	1082	MFV *Ronan Padraig*		Saved boat/rescued 6
1988				
17/02/1988	1082	MFV *Argent*		Escorted vessel
23/03/1988	1082	MFV *Suffolk Crusader*	Man overboard	Search failed
21/05/1988	1082	MFV *Sea Angler*		Others coped
12/06/1988	1082	Small fishing boat		Landed casualty
18/07/1988	1082	Sailing dingy	Capsized	Others coped
23/07/1988	1082	Yacht		Saved boat/rescued 5
10/08/1988	1082	Yacht stranded		Others coped
10/08/1988	1082	MFV *Balaenorta*	Ill man	Landed casualty thereby saving his life
12/11/1988	1082	Fishing vessel	Ill man	Landed casualty

1989				
13/01/1989	1082	Trawler *Big Cat* of Falmouth		Landed a body and put Coast Lifesaving team ashore on Beginish Island
28/01/1989	1082	Trawler *Zorreo Zware*	Injured man	Landed casualty
23/02/1989	1082	Trawler *Roustel*	Ill man	Put doctor on board. Doctor and unconscious man airlifted from vessel
23/06/1989	1082		Distress flares	Search failed
14/06/1989	1108	Trawler *Luas Na Mara*		Landed vessel
02/07/1989	1108	FV *Salamander*	Injured man	Landed casualty
16/07/1989	1108		Distress flares	Search failed
21/07/1989	1108	MFV *Lios Dairbhre*		Others coped
22/07/1989	1108	Persons stranded on rocks at Waterville		Others coped
29/09/1989	1082	FV *Vasslig Kikvidze*	Injured man	Landed casualty
03/11/1989	1082	Persons swept off Culloo Rocks on Valentia		Search failed
14&15/11/ 1989	1082			Landed two bodies of above
04/11/1989	1082	FV *Faithful*		Others coped
07/11/1989	1082		Persons overdue on Blasket Islands	Picked up by MV *Silver Fern*
01/12/1989	1082	FV *Westerly*	Aground on Perch Rock	Took off some crew. Stood by until vessel refloated

Services 1990–2008

Date	LB	Casualty	Cause	Assessment
06/01/1990	1082	MFV *Sea Fisher* of Tralee	Leak	Others coped
25/01/1990	1082	FV *Stella Orion* of Fleetwood	Ill man	Landed 1

30/01/1990	1082	FV *Garadoza*	Stranding	Others coped. Seas 20-2 metres
01/01/1990	1082	FV *Garadoza*	Man overboard	Others coped
04/05/1990	1082	MFV *Three Brothers* of Dingle	Leak	Others coped
31/05/1990	1082	Small boat with outboard	Machinery failure	Others coped
18/06/1990	1082	MFV *Eilis* of Tralee	Machinery failure	Landed craft
07/08/1990	1082	MFV *Catriona*	Man overboard	Search failed
31/08/1990	1082	Inflatable power craft	Machinery failure	Landed vessel
13/10/1990	1082	Rowing boat	Adverse conditions	Others coped
1991				
04/03/1991	1082	MFV *Moon*	Wind	Landed
09/03/1991	1082		Body in sea	Landed
17/03/1991	1082	MFV *Swanella* of Hull	Ill man	Landed
30/03/1991	1082	Yacht *Gipsy* of Limerick	Position unsure	Landed
01/04/1991	1082	Sailing dinghy	Capsize	Others coped
25/05/1991	1082	FV *Paula Dee*	Machinery failure	Landed
06/06/1991	1082	*Petit Fanch* Portmagee	Machinery failure	Landed boat and 3
12/06/1991	1082	Sail yacht catamaran	Multi hull stranded	Others coped
11/07/1991	1082	*Squirrel* of Galway	ill man	Escorted
14/07/1991	1082	Sail board		Others coped
17/07/1991	1082	Power boat		Others coped
21/07/1991	1082	Rowing boat		Others coped
06/08/1991	1082	Inflatable dinghy	Over due	Stood by
13/09/1991	1082	MFV *Rosebud* of Tralee		Saved boat and 2
18/09/1991	1082	Yacht *Peace*		Landed craft and 1
24/09/1991	1082	Helicopter of Celtic Helicopters	Crash	Others coped
24/10/1991	1082	Petit Fanch Portmagee		Landed craft

29/10/1991	1082	Yacht *Wings of the Morning* of Boston		Saved vessel and 2
04/12/1991	1082	Yacht *Wings of the Morning* of Boston		Landed craft and 2
1992				
02/03/1992	1082	Blue sail dinghy		Saved craft and landed 3
10/05/1992	1082		Canoes overdue	False alarm
31/05/1992	1082	Helicopter	Helicopter in sea	Others coped
16/07/1992	1082	MFV *Brigette*		Landed craft and 3
22/07/1992	1082	MFV Fishing Machine		Saved craft and rescued 2
14/08/1992	1082	MV small	Power boat	Others coped
17/08/1992	1082	18 foot small boat		Others coped
10/09/1992	1082	FV small rubber duck		Others coped
14/09/1992	1082	Small power boat	Adverse conditions	Landed craft and 1
21/12/1992	1082	MFV *Monti-Marie* of Spain	Stranded	Landed craft
1993				
02/01/1993	1082		Distress signal	Hoax confirmed
03/03/1993	1082	MFV *Castor et Polleaux*	Fouled propeller	Landed craft
30/03/1993	1082	Russian factory ship *Tarkiluch*		False alarm
06/04/1993	1082	Yacht *Green Goose*	Sails failed	Others coped
14/04/1993	1082	MFV *Roving swan* of Dingle	Machinery failure	Landed craft
24/04/1993	1082	MFV *Prospective* of Dublin	Machinery failure	Landed craft and 5
28/04/1993	1082	MFV *Beal Bocht* of Tralee	Machinery failure	Landed craft and 4
28/04/1993	1082	MFV *Prospective* of Dublin		Landed craft and 5
19/05/1993	1082	Skelligs Rock	Person injured	Took out doctor. Person landed

05/06/1993	1082		Distress signal	Search failed
12/06/1993	1082	MFV *Skua*	Swamping	Others coped
30/06/1993	1082	Dinghy	Overdue	Others coped
06/07/1993	1082	MFV *Silent Seas*	Machinery failure	Landed craft
01/08/1993	1082	Yacht *Les Bis* of France	Adverse conditions	Others coped
01/08/1993	1082	Pleasure boat	Fouled propeller	Landed craft and 3
01/08/1993	1082	Small fishing vessel	Overdue	Escorted
03/08/1993	1082	Small power boat	Stranding	Others coped
08/08/1993	1082	Cruiser *Sarah AnnCab*	Fouled propeller	Landed craft and 3
09/08/1993	1082	Yacht *Geraldine* of Dingle	Stranding	Landed craft
20/08/1993	1082	FV Small fishing vessel	May be trouble	False alarm
20/08/1993	1082	Small cabin cruiser	Overdue	Others coped, Ex RNLB *Rowland Watts* assisted in search
25/08/1993	1082	MFV *Luas Na Mara*	Machinery failure	Saved boat and 1
12/09/1993	1082	FV *Dumnonia* of Spain	Machinery failure	Saved vessel and 12
05/10/1993	1082	FV *Ocean Wanderer* of Tralee	Fouled propeller	Saved boat and 3
14/11/1993	1082		Distress flares/ Adverse conditions	Others coped
19/12/1993	1082		Distress flares	False alarm
1994				
24/02/1994	1082	MV small ferryboat	Capsize	Others coped
10/03/1994	1082	FV *Pascalanza Uno* of Britain	Ill man	Landed casualty
17/04/1994	1082	Sailing dinghy	Capsize	Saved boat
03/06/1994	1082	MV *Snabh* of Tralee	Others coped	
13/06/1994	1082	MFV *Una Allen* of Castletownbere	Fouled propeller	Brought in craft and 5

07/07/1994 (Hibernia)	1150	MFV Marbe Tres	Fouled propeller	Saved boat and 4
07/08/1994	1150	Yacht Quan Yen of Canada	Machinery failure	Saved boat and 1
22/08/1994	1150	Arnold Juan of Castletownbere	Fouled propeller	Saved boat and rescued 3
07/09/1994	1150	Yacht Dotty Dee of Canada	Sail failure	Escorted
11/09/1994	1150		Person fallen from cliff	Gave help
14/09/1994	1150	MFV Strathair of Dingle	Machinery failure	Saved boat and rescued 5
27/09/1994	1150	MFV Kvalholm of Dingle	Leak	Escorted casualty
12/10/1994	1150	Yacht Trembo-Too of Dublin	Position unsure	Escorted casualty
29/12/1994 (Margaret Frances Love)	1082	MFV Delores Cadrechaof Vigo Spain		Crewman landed
1995				
13/01/1995	1082	MFV Cornelis Ferdinand of Tralee	Swamping	Stood by
24/02/1995	1082		Distress signal	False alarm
01/03/1995	1082	Annuction Rivero of Vigo	Leak	Others coped
24/03/1995	1082	FV Undaunted II of Dingle	Fouled propeller	Brought in craft and 5
27/03/1995	1082	MFV Capall Ban of Galway	Fouled propeller	Brought in craft and 5
18/04/1995	1082	Canoes	Overdue	False alarm
23/04/1995	1082	MFV Orion of Castletownbere	Fouled propeller	Brought in craft and 5
03/06/1995	1082	Semi-rigid inflatable of Dublin	Machinery failure	Saved boat and rescued 9
04/06/1995	1082	Skelligs Rock	Injured person fallen from cliff	Others coped
27/06/1995	1082	Yacht Witch Hazel of Cork	Position unsure	Brought in boat and 4
25/07/1995	1082	Jemaleen of Kinsale		Landed craft and 5
26/07/1995	1082	Skelligs Rocks	Fire in buildings	7 persons brought in

10/08/1995	1082	FV 26 foot fishing vessel	Fouled propeller	Others coped
15/08/1995	1082	MFV *Castor et Pollux* of Tralee	Machinery failure	Brought in boat and 4 52.05N 10.56W
14/09/1995	1082	*EIRPB*	Distress signal	False alarm 52.04N 10.27W
15/09/1995	1082		Alleged bomb scare on aircraft	Cancelled/No launch
27/09/1995	1082	MFV *An Tearaght* of Dingle	Machinery failure	Escorted vessel 51.98N 10.35W
13/10/1995	1082	MFV *Hummer* of Sneem	Machinery failure	Others coped 51.76N 09.93W
12/12/1995	1082	MFV *Patos Wish* of Tralee	Fouled propeller	Brought in craft and 5 51.92N 10.96W
1996				
31/01/1996	1082	FV *Equaliser*	Machinery failure	Brought in craft and 2 51.38N 10.10W
15/03/1996	1082	FV *Johanna Maria*	Machinery failure	Escorted vessel 51.45N 10.36W
28/03/1996	1082	FV *Ard Fionnbharr*	Fouled propeller	Brought in craft and 3 51.78N 10.71W
29/03/1996	1082	FV *Marber Therese*	Fouled propeller	Brought in craft and 4 51.40N 10.27W
03/05/1996	1082	FV *Staronia*	Fouled propeller	Brought in craft and 4 51.41N 10.47W
06/05/1996	1082	UnknownPower boat	Overdue	False alarm Westcove/Kenmare area
07/05/1996	1082	FV *Fionnbhar*	Fouled propeller	Brought in craft and 4 51.48N 10.62W
10/05/1996	1082	FV *Emma Elizabeth*	Leak/swamping	Others coped 51.34N 10.12W
29/05/1996	1082	FV *Nozi Dei*	Fouled propeller	Brought in craft and 3 51.42N10.43W
30/05/1996	1082	Yacht *Boney*	Drags anchor	Others coped Kenmare Bay
30/05/1996	1082	MV *Arklow Abbey*		Escorted casualty NES4 miles NW of Valentia
02/06/1996	1082	FV *Ocean Flower*	Machinery failure	Brought in craft and 2 Bolus Head
10/06/1996	1082	Yacht *Wind Flower*	Machinery failure	Brought in craft and 3 51.12N 10.28W

20/06/1996	1082	FV *Beal Insemall*	Machinery failure	Landed craft and 8 51.94N 10.36W
21/06/1996	1082	FV *Janet Ann*	Man overboard	Search failed 51.29N 10.22W
24/06/1996	1082	Yacht *Big Ears*	Ill man	Landed 1 51.42N 10.34W
24/06/1996	1082	Rubber dinghy	Adverse conditions	Rescued 1 52.04N 10.13W
04/07/1996	1082	FV *Duella*	Fouled propeller	Brought in craft and 1 3 miles NE of Skelligs
23/08/1996	1082	Bather Inch beach		False alarm
28/08/1996	1082	FV *Ocean Wanderer* of Tralee	Fouled propeller	Landed craft and 2 51.92N 10.29W
09/09/1996	1082	MV *Emily Frances*	Man overboard	Landed a body 51.63N 10.47W
23/10/1996	1082	*Bylgta* of Dingle	Steering failure	Others coped 51.84N 09.69W
18/11/1996 (*John and Margaret Doig*)	1218	Dredger *Germaine* of Arklow	Adverse conditions	Escorted casualty
27/11/1996	1218	Tug *Buffin*	Fouled propeller	Stood by 51.52N 10.25W
02/12/1996	1218	MFV *Tournalet* of Concarnau, France	Fouled propeller	Saved boat and rescued 9 52.04N 10.51W
17/12/1996	1218	*Orka* of Dingle	Machinery failure	Landed craft and 3 52.09N1 0.51W
1997				
23/01/1997	1218	MFV *Shannon* of Dingle	Machinery failure	Escorted casualty
09/03/1997	1218	MFV *Exodus* of Castletownbere	Leak/ swamping	Others coped
14/04/1997	1218	MFV *Laochra Beara* of Castletownbere	Leak/ swamping	Others coped
19/04/1997	1218	Motor cruiser	Machinery failure	Others coped
20/04/1997	1218	FV *Iolar Na Mara* of Tralee	Fouled propeller	Brought in craft and 3
23/04/1997	1218	MV *Skellig Dawn* of Dingle	Machinery failure	Saved craft and rescued 2

14/05/1997	1218	MFV *Noreen Juliet* of Tralee	Machinery failure	Brought in craft and 3
13/06/1997	1218	Rowing boat	Man overboard	Landed 1
20/06/1997	1218	MFV *Dakkar* of Dingle	Stranding	Gave help
13/07/1997	1218	Canoes	Overdue	False alarm
17/07/1997	1218	*Isac II* of Dublin	Machinery failure	Brought in craft and 9
22/07/1997	1218	MFV *Puffin* of Dumfries, Scotland	Leak/ swamping	Saved boat and 3
30/07/1997	1218		Persons washed off rocks/ Persons fallen from cliff	Saved 2
31/07/1997	1218	Twice	Persons missing	Searches failed
01/08/1997	1218	Four times	Persons missing	Searches failed
02/08/1997	1218		Persons missing	Search failed
02/08/1997	1218		Persons missing	Landed a body
02/08/1997	1218	Bathers	5 swimmers missing	Others coped
05/08/1997	1218	MFV *Hakien* of Spain	Ill man	Landed 1
14/08/1997	1218	MFV *Blue Chip* of Limerick	Leak/ swamping	Gave help
17/08/1997	1218	MFV *Castor et Polloux* of Portmagee	Leak/ swamping	Saved boat and rescued 2
17/08/1997	1218	MFV *Early Bird* of Tralee	Machinery failure	Landed craft and 6
20/08/1997	1218	MFV *Heather Valley* of Tralee	Machinery failure	Landed craft and 7
23/09/1997	1218	MFV *Janet Ann* of Castletownbere	Ill man	Others coped
03/10/1997	1218	MFV *Ard Eireann* of Castletownbere	Leak/ swamping	Gave help
23/10/1997	1218	Open small boat	Overdue	Search failed

24/10/1997	1218	16ft boat with outboard motor	Overdue	Landed body
23/12/1997	1218		Person in water	Others coped
1998				
25/01/1998	1218	FV *Rosses Morn* of Castletownbere	Ill man	Person brought in
17/02/1998	1218	FV *Marber Terease* of Tralee	Fouled propeller	Brought in craft and 4
25/02/1998	1218	FV *Ard Fionbharr* of Dingle	Fouled propeller	Brought in craft and 4
25/02/1998	1218	FV *Strathcairn* of Dingle	Steering failed	Others coped
24/03/1998	1218	FV *Rose Crest* of Tralee	Fouled propeller	Gave help
11/04/1998	1218	Yacht *The Old Lady*	Machinery failure	Others coped
14/04/1998	1218	MV *Thundercrest* of Tralee	Machinery failure	Rescued 10 people
03/05/1998	1218	MV *Sea Quest*	Machinery failure	Brought in craft and 7
05/05/1998	1218	MFV *Strathclyde* of Dingle	Machinery failure	Brought in craft and 4
09/06/1998	1218	Yacht *Sherpa Bell of Isle of Wight*	Dragging anchor	Brought in craft and 2 people
12/06/1998	1218	*The Old Lady* power boat	Machinery failure	Others coped
22/06/1998	1218	Yacht *Army New Age* of Dublin	Sail failure	Saved yacht and rescued 12 people
08/07/1998	1218	FV *Spailpin Fanach* of Tralee	Machinery failure	Others coped
28/07/1998	1218	Yacht *Topaz* of Dublinft	Steering failed	Brought in craft and 2
29/07/1998	1218	FV *Ard Eireann* of Castletownbere	Fouled propeller	Brought in craft and 3
01/08/1998	1218	Yacht *Lechwee* of Kinsale	Fouled propeller	Landed craft and 6 1 mile west of Cromwell's Point
02/08/1998	1218	FV *Marie H* English	Ill man	Brought in 2 people 52.03N 14.10W
07/08/1998	1218	Diver	Missing	Gave help

12/08/1998	1218	FV *Donegal* of Tralee	Machinery failure	Brought in craft and 4 Inch beach
13/08/1998	1218	FV *Jerdemar* of Tralee	Position unsure	Others coped Skelligs
26/08/1998	1218	Sail board	Adverse conditions	Others coped 51.83N 10.22W
17/10/1998	1218		Distress signal	False alarm
01/12/1998	1218	FV *Castor et Pollux* of Tralee	Fouled propeller	Brought in craft and 3 51.57N 10.59W
1999				
17/01/1999	1218		Red flares	Search failed Bray Head area
11/02/1999	1218	MV *Altair* of Dingle	Fire	Saved craft Dingle Bay
19/04/1999	1218	Yacht *Enterprise* of Kilrush	Sail failure	Saved craft and rescued 5 2.03N10.56W
28/04/1999	1218		Persons swept away/Persons cut off	Others coped Kenmare Bay
04/06/1999	1218		Man washed off rocks	Brought in one person Inis TuaisceartBlaskets
04/06/1999	1218		Persons missing	Assembly/no launchFalse alarm Castlemaine
13/06/1999	1218	*River Dancer*	Leak/ swamping	Others coped Portmagee harbour
28/06/1999	1218	FV *Ocean Reaper* of Dingle	Ill man	One person brought in Dingle Bay
09/08/1999	1218	FV *Skelligs Light* of Dublin	Ill man	One person brought in north of Valentia
19/10/1999	1218	*Rysa Lass* tug/ barge	Machinery failure	Landed craft and 2 west of Lamb Island
24/10/1999	1218	Containers		False alarm 2 miles off Slea Head
30/10/1999	1218	FV *Invension*	Leak/ swamping	Other coped 60 miles west of Valentia
07/11/1999	1218	FV *Celestial Dawn*	Machinery failure	Brought in craft and 7 51.45N 11.01W
25/11/1999 (EIRPB)	1150		Distress signal	False alarm 51.27N 10.49W
25/11/1999	1150	FV *Sant*	Position unsure	Escorted casualty Approach to Valentia harbour

01/12/1999	1150	FV *Eoin Aoife* of Cork	Position unsure	Others coped 51.41N 10.07W
22/12/1999	1150		Flares seen in Dingle Bay	False alarm
2000				
17/01/2000	1150	FV *St Jervaise*	Leak/ swamping	Gave help 52.14.3N 11.03.1W
19/03/2000	1150	FV *Dernaline*	Fouled propeller	Landed craft and 4 52.10N 11.16W
05/04/2000	1150	FV *Spailpin Fanach*	Ill crewman	Gave help 2.10N 11.28W
17/04/2000	1150	MV *Moira Michelle*	Steering failure	Brought in craft and 1 2 miles NW of Cromwells Point Lighthouse
20/04/2000	1150	FV *St Jervaise*	Fouled propeller	Stood by Near Beginish Island
23/04/2000	1150	20 foot open boat. No name	Machinery failure	Landed craft and 4 3 miles NW of Coonanna
13/05/2000	1150	*Tearaght*	Ill man	Landed casualty Tearaght Island
13/05/2000	1150	Diving boat. No name	Leak/ swamping	Landed craft and 6 Puffin Island
11/06/200	1218		Person threatening to jump from cliff	Stood by Culloo
19/06/2000	1218	Children	Reported missing	False alarm Rossbeigh Beach
26/06/2000	1218	Yacht *Couilles De Chien*	Steering failure	Brought in craft and landed 1 51.58N 10.32W
30/06/2000	1218	FV *Ardent* of Cork	Ill man	Landed casualty 52.33N 12.08W
19/07/2000	1218	*Ocean Star*	Machinery failure	Brought in craft and 3 ½ mile NNEof Dolus Head
27/07/2000	1218	*Celtic Star* Large power boat	Machinery failure	Others coped 2 miles NW of Puffin Island
02/08/2000	1218	Yacht *Freedom* of *Norwich*	Machinery failure	Others coped 51.46 No9.54W
09/08/2000	1218	FV *Ocean Reaper*	Fouled propeller	Brought in craft and 5 51.57N10.45W

24/08/2000	1218	FV *Carberry Maid*	Fouled propeller	Brought in craft and 2 1 mile east of Dolus Head
28/08/2000	1218	FV *Glenravel*	Machinery failure	Brought in craft and 7 3 miles west of Dolus Head
31/08/2000	1218	FV *Castor et Pollux*	Fouled propeller	Landed craft and 5 51.62N 10.35W
31/08/2000	1218	FV *Castor et Pollux*	Dragging anchor	Gave help Valentia harbour
10/09/2000	1218	FV *Ard Eireann*	Fire	Others coped 51.42N 10.15W
05/10/2000	1218	Object–EIRPB transmitting	Object reported	Search failed
05/10/2000	1218		Flare distress signal	False alarm Ventry harbour
11/10/2000	1218		Distress signal	False alarm
25/11/2000	1218	Small power boat, no name	Man overboard	Rescued 1
2001				
21/01/2001	1218	MFV *Galaxia* of Spain	Fire	Landed 10 50.02N12.05W
11/03/2001 (*Hyman Winstone*)	1067	FV *Myrdoma*	Ill man	Landed 1
12/03/2001	1067	FV *Simplan*	Ill man	Landed 1 3 miles NW of Cromwells Point
23/05/2001	1150	MV *Flying Horse*	Leak/ swamping	Brought in craft and 1 ¼ mile NE of Skelligs
22/06/2001	1150	Large tanker *Forth Fisher*	Man overboard	Search failed 51.33N 10.24W
30/06/2001	1150		Flares distress signal	False alarm Slea Head
17/02/2001	1218	FV *Blue Boy*	Machinery failure	Others coped Smerwick harbour
29/07/2001	1218	*Lady Helena* small power boat	Position unsure	Escorted casualty 52.05N 10.02Wo
04/09/2001	1218	*Joan of Arc* angling vessel	Machinery failure	Brought in craft and 8 Foher Cliffs
09/09/2001	1218	FV *Driocht Na Mara*	Machinery failure	Landed craft and 5 51.49N 19.35W

02/10/2001	1218		Persons missing	False alarm
03/10/2001	1218		Persons missing	False alarm Foher Cliffs
12/10/2001	1218	FV *Regina Ponti*	Ill man	Brought in 1 person 51.52N 10.46W
2002				
26/01/2002	1218	FV *Skelligs Dawn*	Machinery failure	Escorted casualty 51.55N 10.36W
28/01/2002	1218	FV *Skelligs Dawn*	Stranding	Landed craft and 14 Near Renard Point
02/02/2002	1218	FV *Celestial Dawn*	Stranding/ Aground at Dingle harbour entrance	Gave help
02/02/2002	1218	FV large Spanish trawler. (No name)	May be trouble sheltering near Blaskets	False Alarm
30/03/2002	1218	Persons missing		Others coped Inch Beach
12/04/2002	1218		Distress flares	False alarm outside Dingle harbour
13/04/2002	1218	*Marian* power boat	Machinery failure	Brought in craft and 2 50.01N 10.28W
02/05/2002	1218	*Marian* power boat	Machinery failure	Brought in craft and 2 1 mile west of Bray Head
04/05/2002	1218	FV *Kopanas*	Stranding	Escorted casualty Cloghavallig Rocks
08/05/2002	1218		Persons missing	Search failed
10/05/2002	1218	FV *Fidelma*	Stranding/ aground	Landed 4 people at Inishnabro Island
12/05/2002	1218	8 metre rib open power boat. No name	Fire	Brought in 6 people 1 mile west of the Great Blasket Island
24/05/2002	1218	FV Magayant	Fouled propeller	Escorted casualty 2 miles west of Dingle
26/05/2002	1218	Bather		False alarm White Strand
12/07/2002	1218	*Marian* large open power	Machinery failure	Brought in craft and 4 Entrance to Valentia at Portmagee

18/07/2002	1218	FV *Gannett*	Machinery failure	Brought in craft and 2 3 miles north of Valentia
31/07/2002	1218	BFV *Dinah*	Machinery failure	Gave help Bray Head
02/08/2002	1218	Yacht *Snug*	Stranding going ashore	Brought in craft and 3 Wireless Point
06/08/2002	1218	*Iolar Na Mara* angling vessel	Steering failure	Brought in 5 and landed craft Off Culloo
08/08/2002 (*Volunteer Spirit*)	1254	FV *Cosantoir Bradan*	Adverse conditions	52.09N 10.38W
11/08/2002	1254	Yatch. No name	Leak/ swamping	Others coped Ventry harbour
11/08/2002	1254	*Merci 5* sail yacht	Sail failure	Saved boat and rescued 6 52.10N 10.35W
11/08/2002	1254	*El Dorada* sail yacht	Stranding	Others coped Westcove Kenmare River
17/08/2002	1254		Persons missing	False alarm Beginish Island
11/12/2002	1218	FV *Naomh Derarca*	Fouled propeller	Landed craft and 3 52.13N 10.24W
2003				
14/01/2003	1218		Distress signal	False alarm
17/02/2003	1218	*Jeanie Johnston* sail training vessel	Adverse conditions	Gave help west of Wireless Point
26/02/2003	1218	FV *Westella*	Ill man	Landed 1 51.5N 10.38W
07/04/2003	1218		Distress signal	False alarm
07/05/2003	1218		Person in water	Landed a body
09/06/2003	1218	*Eagle III* open power boat	Machinery failure	Landed craft and 11 Coastguard Patch off Dolus Head
11/06/2003	1218	FV *Pato's Wish*	Machinery failure	Brought in craft and 3 51.55N 10.39W
09/07/2003	1218	Yacht *Happy Days*	Position unsure	Landed craft and 1 St Finian's Bay
12/07/2003	1218	Yacht *Supple*		Brought in craft and 3 north of Lighthouse
14/07/2003	1218	FV *La Mesange*	Fouled propeller	Brought in craft and 6 52.18N 10.44W

19/07/2003	1218	Yacht *Bel-Ami*	Machinery failure	Landed craft and 3 1 mile NW Cromwell Lighthouse
26/07/2003	1218		Diver missing	Others coped
08/08/2003	1218	FV *Ocean Star II*	Machinery failure	Brought in craft and 3 2 miles west of Bolus Head
23/08/2003	1218	Power boat *Orca II*	Fouled propeller	Brought in craft and 3 51.52N 10.26W
03/09/2003	1218	Power boat *Shady H*	Machinery failure	Brought in craft and 4 1 mile off Dolus Head
06/09/2003	1218	Diving boat *Kittiwake*	Machinery failure	Brought in craft and 6 Basalt cliff at Beginish
15/09/2003	1218	FV large *Aelindrew*	Fouled propeller	Brought in craft and 5 51.56N 10.20W
2004				
30/03/2004	1218	FV *Grainne Marie*	Machinery failure	Brought in craft and 2 Coastguard Patch
12/04/2004	1218		Diver missing	Gave help
16/04/2004	1218	FV *Ocean Glory*	Machinery failure	Brought in craft and 1 Foileye Point, Kells
02/05/2004	1218		Diver missing	Others coped
06/06/2004	1218	*Framaria* large power boat	Machinery failure	Brought in craft and 4 52.05N 10.29W
08/06/2004	1218	FV *Ocean Wanderer*	Machinery failure	Brought in craft and 2 Culloo
12/06/2004	1218	Yacht and aux. *Kerry Gannet*	Fouled propeller	Gave help 1 mile west of Dolus Head
05/07/2004	1218	Yacht and aux. *Star of the Sea*	Machinery failure	Brought in craft and 8 1 mile north of Teareaght
08/07/2004	1218	FV *Phoenix*	Machinery failure	Brough in craft and 2 Caherciveen River
12/07/2004	1218	FV *Grainne Marie*	Machinery failure	Brought in craft and 2 north of Bray Head
18/07/2004	1218	FV *Roisin*	Machinery failure	Brought in craft and 2 1 mile north of Cromwell Point
23/07/2004	1218	*Silver Fisher II* power boat	Fouled propeller	Brought in craft and 3 52.12N 10.23W
07/08/2004	1218	Diving boat. No name	Machinery failure	Bought in craft and 4 52.05N 10.34W

12/08/2004	1218	FV *St Gabrali*	Fouled propeller	Stood by NE side of Puffin Island
09/09/2004	1218	FV *Nicolia*	Machinery failure	Brought in craft and 5 Culloo
28/09/2004	1218	FV Spailpin *Fanach*	Fire	Landed 3 51.46N 10.50W
13/10/2004	1218	1 person kite board		Others coped Inch strand
05/11/2004	1218	FV *Noreen Bawn*	Fouled propeller	Escorted casualty Blasket Sound
07/11/2004	1218	FV *Ard Alainnarge*	Fouled propeller	Brought in craft and 3 51.36N 10.37 W
26/11/2004	1218	FV *Nicola V*	Fouled propeller	Brought in craft and 1 Dingle Bay
03/12/2004	1218	FV *Grainne Marie*	Fouled propeller	Brought in craft and 2 51.46N 10.88W
04/12/200	41218	FV small. No name	Overdue	False alarm Dingle Bay
17/12/2004	1218	FV *Ornalomar*	Ill man	Landed casualty 51.56N 10.20W
2005				
10/03/2005	1218	FV *Sweet Waters*	Machinery failure	Brought in craft and 1 51.59N 10.14W
19/03/2005	1218	Diving boat. No name	Machinery failure	Brought in craft and 8 Lough Kay
06/04/2005	1218	FV *Guiding Star*	Stranding	Escorted vessel 52.10N 10.88W
18/04/2005	1218	*Sioux* Angling boat	Machinery failure	Brought in craft and 11 51.48N 10.28W
01/05/2005	1218	FV *Helios*	Fouled propeller	Brought in craft and 5
30/05/2005	1218	Passenger vessel. No name	Fouled propeller	Brought in craft and 1
13/06/2005	1218	Yacht. No name	Machinery failed	Brought in craft and 2
26/06/2005	1218			False alarm
15/07/2005	1218		Bather drowning	False alarm
17/07/2005	1218	Small power boat. No name	Machinery failure	Brought in craft and 3
04/08/2005	1218	Fishing vessel. No name	Machinery failure	Brought in craft and 3
15/08/2005	1218			False alarm

15/08/2005	1218	Power boat. No name	Machinery failure	Brought in craft and 3
18/08/2005	1218	Angling vessel. No name	Machinery failure	Brought in craft and 8
29/08/2005	1218	FV *Spailpin Fanach*	Fire	Landed 4
08/10/2005	1218		Animal in trouble	Gave help
15/10/2005	1218	Power boat. No name	Leak/ swamping	Saved boat and landed 3
11/11/2005	1218	*Hannibal II*	Machinery failure	Others coped
22/11/2005	1218	FV *Grainne Marie*	Fouled propeller	Brought in craft and 1
2006				
22/01/2006	1218	FV *Pilgrim Light*	Leaks or swamping	Gave help 51.52N 10.37W
21/03/2006	1218	FV Girl Julie	Machinery failure	Brought in vessel and 3 51.43N 10.24 W
26/03/2006 (*Volunteer Spirit*)	1254	*Pors Piron*	Stranding or grounding	Brought in 4 mouth of Dingle harbour
31/03/2006	1254		Person fallen from cliff	Unsuccessful search Ballinskelligs
01/04/2006	1254		Dead body	Unsuccessful search Ballinskelligs
02/04/2006	1254		Dead body	Unsuccessful search Ballinskelligs
10/05/2006	1254	FV *Gannet*	Machinery failure	Recovered vessel and brought in 1 52.02N10.33W
26/05/2006	1254	FV large. No name	Grounding	Brought in 4
13/07/2006	1218	*Sinead* large open power boat	Machinery failure	Recovered vessel and brought in 3 52.01N10.37W
19/07/2006	1218	Jet ski		Others coped Rossbeigh Beach
02/08/2006	1218	FV *Marber Therese*	Fouled propeller or impeller	Recovered vessel and brought in 4 4 miles west of Bray Head
03/08/2006	1218	FV *Beal Inse*	Leaks or swamping	Recovered vessel and brought in 2 Cromwell Point

20/08/2006	1218	An old hull adrift for a long period of time	Capsize	Others coped Portmagee harbour
09/09/2006	1218	Sailboard	Overdue	Others coped Rossbeigh Beach
01/10/2006	1218	*Kindred Spirit* large open power boat	Machinery failure	Recovered craft and brought in 1 52.02N10.26W
2007				
07/02/2007	1218	FV *Joseph*	Ill man	Landed casualty Skelligs
14/02/2007	1218	FV *Emma Lou*	Machinery failure	Recovered craft and brought in 2 Valentia harbour
02/03/2007	1218	FV *Emma Lou*	Steering failure	Recovered craft and brought in 2 Caherciveen River
17/03/2007	1218	FV *Manuel Laura*	Ill man	Landed casualty Blasket Islands
10/04/2007	1218	Passenger vessel. No name	Leaks or swamping	Others coped Dingle harbour
11/04/2007	1218	*West Sailor* Tanker	Machinery failure	Gave help Tralee Bay
20/04/2007	1218	Small fishing boat	Stranding or grounding	Others coped south side of Valentia
04/05/2007	1218	FV *Marber Therese*	Machinery failure	Recovered vessel and brought in 3 10 miles west of Bray Head
13/05/2007	1218	*Mary Francis* angling vessel	Machinery failure	Recovered vessel and brought in 10 Wireless Point
19/05/2007	1218	Yacht with aux. engine. No name	Stranding or grounding	Others coped Smerwick harbour
01/06/2007	1218	Passenger vessel. No name	Machinery failure	Recovered vessel and brought in 2 Skelligs Rock
06/06/2007	1218	Bather	Person missing	Others coped Blaskets Sound
09/06/2007	1218	Yacht *Imaraguen* with aux. engine	Sail failure or dismasting	Recovered vessel and brought in 2 75 miles north-west of Valentia
04/07/2007	1218	Yacht *Enya* with aux. engine	Adverse conditions	Gave help. Approach to Valentia harbour

13/07/2007	1218	Skelligs Rock	Person injured	Landed casualty Skelligs
13/07/2007	1218	Cliff climber	Drowning	Unsuccessful search Wireless Point
14/07/2007	1218	Cliff climber	Drowning	Unsuccessful search Wireless Point
15/07/2007	1218	Cliff climber	Missing	Unsuccessful search Wireless Point
16/07/2007	1218		Person in water	Resolved unaided
04/08/2007	1218	Yacht *Jaconel* with aux. engine	Machinery failure	Recovered craft and brought in 3 1 mile north of Dolus Head
05/08/2007	1218	Yacht *Silent Years* with aux. engine	Stranding or grounding	Gave help Beginish Bar
09/08/2007	1218	*Jeanie Johnston* Passenger vessel	Ill man	Landed casualty off Skelligs
01/10/2007	1218	FV *Rose Crest*	Machinery failure	Recovered craft and brought in 2 2 miles north of Skelligs
12/10/2007	1218	Vessel thought to be in trouble	Distress flares	Hoax confirmed
14/0/2007	1218		Distress signal	False alarm
2008				
22/01/2008	1218	FV *Fletcha*	Injured man	Landed casualty at Skelligs
07/02/2008	1218	FV *Caoimhuala*	Machinery failure	Brought in craft and landed 5 at Dingle off Blaskets
26/02/2008	1218	Object in the sea	Floating container	False alarm between Scarriff and Hogs Head
20/03/2008	1218		Flares	False alarm at Beal Tra
27/03/2008	1218	Yacht *The Silver Dipper*	Adverse conditions	Saved boat and rescued 4 north–west of the Blaskets
28/03/2008	1218		Red flares	False alarm White Strand/Cahirciveen River
14/04/2008	1218	Yacht *Kerry Gannet*	Fouled propeller	Brought in craft and 1 south of Bray Head

15/04/2008	1218	FV *Petit Franch*	Machinery failure	Brought in craft and 3 north west of the Blaskets
07/05/2008	1218	Power boat	Boarding boat	Others coped
08/05/2008	1218		Missing person	Search failed Rossbeigh Beach
14/05/2008	1218	Yacht *Euronav* Belgica	Fuel shortage	Brought in craft and 2 50 miles west of Skelligs
19/05/2008	1218	*Flying Horse* passenger vessel	Machinery failure	Brought in craft and 12 between Skelligs and Ballinskelligs
06/06/2008	1218	*Nicholisa* Power boat	Fuel shortage	Brought in craft and 2 off Valentia
20/06/2008	1218	FV *Celtic Quest*	Required assistance	Brought in craft and 5
21/06/2008	1218	FV *Conquest*	Requested assistance	Brought in craft and 4
07/07/2008	1218	Sailing dinghy	Capsized	Resolved unaided
14/07/2008	1218	Yacht *Oleron*	Could not enter Dingle harbour	Escorted vessel
07/08/2008	1218	*Moment of Madness* power boat	Required assistance	Escorted vessel
16/08/2008	1218	Power boat	Vessel in difficulty	Brought in craft and 1 west of Inch Beach
18/08/2008	1218	Rowing boat	Upturned vessel	False alarm Foileye Head
30/09/2008	1218		Person in sea	Landed a body Culloo Valentia
30/09/2008	1218	Yacht *Magnolia*	Adverse conditions	Brought in craft and 3 Valentia harbour entrance
26/10/2008	1218		Person fallen from cliff	Saved 1 life Culloo Valentia

Valentia Lifeboat Services Analysis

1970

All Services (including assemblies)	1
Crew Assemblies (no launch)	
Lives Saved	10
Persons Landed	17
Persons Brought In	
Services to Crafts Saved/Landed	1
Successful Services	9
Co-ordinated by Coastguard	0
Non RNLI Lives Lost	1
Persons Injured	0
Hoax/False Alarms	2
Unsuccessful Searches	0
Lifeboat Unable to Complete Service	0
Others Coped	2
To Merchant and Fishing Vessels	5
To Pleasure Craft	2
To People	2
To Other Types of Casualty	3
Property Saved Value	£500
Services by Lifeboat	11
Services with Air Cooperation	1
Services Wind Over Force Seven	5
Services in Darkness	9
Services with Doctor/Auxillary on Board	0
Services Crew Claimed Salvage	0
Lifeboat Hours at Sea	112.7
Crew – Man Hours at Sea	807.7

1971

All Services (including assemblies)	13
Crew Assemblies (no launch)	9
Lives Saved	6
Persons Landed	0
Persons Brought In	0
Services to Crafts Saved/Landed	3
Successful Services	11
Co-ordinated by Coastguard	0
Non RNLI Lives Lost	2
Person' Injured	0

Hoax/False Alarms	1
Unsuccessful Searches	4
Lifeboat Unable to Complete Service	0
Others Coped	3
To Merchant and Fishing Vessels	6
To Pleasure Craft	3
To People	0
To Other Types of Casualty	4
Property Saved Value	£55,000
Services by Lifeboat	13
Services with Air Cooperation	2
Services Wind Over Force Seven	0
Services in Darkness	12
Services with Doctor/Auxillary on Board	0
Services Crew Claimed Salvage	0
Lifeboat Hours at Sea	110.8
Crew – Man Hours at Sea	790.9

1972

All Services (including assemblies)	12
Crew Assemblies (no launch)	0
Lives Saved	23
Persons Landed	1
Persons Brought In	
Services to Crafts Saved/Landed	5
Successful Services	9
Co-ordinated by Coastguard	0
Non RNLI Lives Lost	0
Persons Injured	0
Hoax/False Alarms	1
Unsuccessful Searches	1
Lifeboat Unable to Complete Service	0
Others Coped	2
To Merchant and Fishing Vessels	9
To Pleasure Craft	0
To People	0
To Other Types of Casualty	3
Property Saved Value	£115,000
Services by Lifeboat	12
Services with Air Cooperation	2
Services Wind Over Force Seven	2
Services in Darkness	6

Services with Doctor/Auxillary on Board	0
Services Crew Claimed Salvage	0
Lifeboat Hours at Sea	75
Crew – Man Hours at Sea	530.1

1973

All Services (including assemblies)	9
Crew Assemblies (no launch)	0
Lives Saved	2
Persons Landed	2
Persons Brought In	24
Services to Crafts Saved/Landed	0
Successful Services	7
Co-ordinated by Coastguard	0
Non RNLI Lives Lost	0
Persons Injured	0
Hoax/False Alarms	0
Unsuccessful Searches	1
Lifeboats Unable to Complete Service	0
Others Coped	0
To Merchant and Fishing Vessels	5
To Pleasure Craft	0
To People	1
To Other Types of Casualty	3
Property Saved Value	0
Services by Lifeboat	9
Services with Air Cooperation	3
Services Wind Over Force Seven	0
Services in Darkness	5
Services with Doctor/Auxillary on Board	2
Services Crew Claimed Salvage	0
Lifeboat Hours at Sea	51.2
Crew – Man Hours at Sea	365.7

1974

All Services (including assemblies)	11
Crew Assemblies (no launch)	0
Lives Saved	5
Persons Landed	0
Persons Brought In	0
Services to Crafts Saved/Landed	2
Successful Services	5

Co-ordinated by Coastguard	0
Non RNLI Lives Lost	1
Persons Injured	0
Hoax/False Alarms	1
Unsuccessful Searches	0
Lifeboat Unable to Complete Service	0
Others Coped	5
To Merchant and Fishing Vessels	5
To Pleasure Craft	2
To People	0
To Other Types of Casualty	4
Property Saved Value	£57,500
Services by Lifeboat	11
Services with Air Cooperation	4
Services Wind Over Force Seven	0
Services in Darkness	3
Services with Doctor/Auxillary on Board	1
Services Crew Claimed Salvage	0
Lifeboat Hours at Sea	49
Crew – Man Hours at Sea	326.9

1975

All Services (including assemblies)	7
Crew Assemblies (no launch)	0
Lives Saved	10
Persons Landed	0
Persons Brought In	0
Services to Crafts Saved/Landed	5
Successful Services	6
Co-ordinated by Coastguard	0
Non RNLI Lives Lost	0
Persons Injured	0
Hoax/False Alarms	0
Unsuccessful Searches	0
Lifeboat Unable to Complete Service	0
Others Coped	1
To Merchant and Fishing Vessels	7
To Pleasure Craft	0
To People	0
To Other Types of Casualty	0
Property Saved Value	£207,500
Services by Lifeboat	7

Services with Air Cooperation   0
Services Wind Over Force Seven   0
Services in Darkness   3
Services with Doctor/Auxillary on Board   1
Services Crew Claimed Salvage   0
Lifeboat Hours at Sea   31.3
Crew – Man Hours at Sea   195.9

1976

All Services (including assemblies)   12
Crew Assemblies (no launch)   0
Lives Saved   0
Persons Landed   3
Persons Brought In   0
Services to Crafts Saved/Landed   4
Successful Services   8
Co-ordinated by Coastguard   0
Non RNLI Lives Lost   2
Persons Injured   0
Hoax/False Alarms   1
Unsuccessful Searches   2
Lifeboat Unable to Complete Service   0
Others Coped   2
To Merchant and Fishing Vessels   8
To Pleasure Craft   1
To People   1
To Other Types of Casualty   2
Property Saved Value   £200,000
Services by Lifeboat   12
Services with Air Cooperation   2
Services Wind Over Force Seven   1
Services in Darkness   7
Services with Doctor/Auxillary on Board   1
Services Crew Claimed Salvage   0
Lifeboat Hours at Sea   60.9
Crew – Man Hours at Sea   439.9

1977

All Services (including assemblies)   6
Crew Assemblies (no launch)   0
Lives Saved   0
Persons Landed   0

Persons Brought In	0
Services to Crafts Saved/Landed	3
Successful Services	5
Co-ordinated by Coastguard	0
Non RNLI Lives Lost	0
Persons Injured	0
Hoax/False Alarms	0
Unsuccessful Searches	0
Lifeboat Unable to Complete Service	0
Others Coped	1
To Merchant and Fishing Vessels	3
To Pleasure Craft	1
To People	1
To Other Types of Casualty	1
Property Saved Value	£55,000
Services by Lifeboat	6
Services with Air Cooperation	1
Services Wind Over Force Seven	0
Services in Darkness	5
Services with Doctor/Auxillary on Board	0
Services Crew Claimed Salvage	0
Lifeboat Hours at Sea	30.0
Crew – Man Hours at Sea	209.3

1978

All Services (including assemblies)	10
Crew Assemblies (no launch)	0
Lives Saved	0
Persons Landed	2
Persons Brought In	0
Services to Crafts Saved/Landed	3
Successful Services	5
Co-ordinated by Coastguard	0
Non RNLI Lives Lost	0
Persons Injured	0
Hoax/False Alarms	2
Unsuccessful Searches	1
Lifeboat Unable to Complete Service	0
Others Coped	4
To Merchant and Fishing Vessels	8
To Pleasure Craft	2
To People	0

To Other Types of Casualty	0
Property Saved Value	£60,000
Services by Lifeboat	10
Services with Air Cooperation	0
Services Wind Over Force Seven	1
Services in Darkness	6
Services with Doctor/Auxillary on Board	0
Services Crew Claimed Salvage	0
Lifeboat Hours at Sea	37.9
Crew – Man Hours at Sea	257.9

1979

All Services (including assemblies)	10
Crew Assemblies (no launch)	0
Lives Saved	0
Persons Landed	2
Persons Brought In	0
Services to Crafts Saved/Landed	3
Successful Services	5
Co-ordinated by Coastguard	0
Non RNLI Lives Lost	0
Persons Injured	0
Hoax/False Alarms	2
Unsuccessful Searches	1
Lifeboat Unable to Complete Service	0
Others Coped	4
To Merchant and Fishing Vessels	8
To Pleasure Craft	2
To People	0
To Other Types of Casualty	0
Property Saved Value	£60,000
Services by Lifeboat	10
Services with Air Cooperation	0
Services Wind Over Force Seven	1
Services in Darkness	6
Services with Doctor/Auxillary on Board	0
Services Crew Claimed Salvage	0
Lifeboat Hours at Sea	37.9
Crew – Man Hours at Sea	257.9

1980

All Services (including assemblies)	10

Crew Assemblies (no launch)	0
Lives Saved	8
Persons Landed	0
Persons Brought In	0
Services to Crafts Saved/Landed	4
Successful Services	8
Co-ordinated by Coastguard	0
Non RNLI Lives Lost	0
Persons Injured	0
Hoax/False Alarms	2
Unsuccessful Searches	2
Lifeboat Unable to Complete Service	0
Others Coped	0
To Merchant and Fishing Vessels	5
To Pleasure Craft	3
To People	2
To Other Types of Casualty	0
Property Saved Value	£157,500
Services by Lifeboat	10
Services with Air Cooperation	2
Services Wind Over Force Seven	4
Services in Darkness	9
Services with Doctor/Auxillary on Board	0
Services Crew Claimed Salvage	0
Lifeboat Hours at Sea	67.2
Crew – Man Hours at Sea	451.6

1981

All Services (including assemblies)	3
Crew Assemblies (no launch)	0
Lives Saved	3
Persons Landed	9
Persons Brought In	0
Services to Crafts Saved/Landed	3
Successful Services	3
Co-ordinated by Coastguard	0
Non RNLI Lives Lost	0
Persons Injured	0
Hoax/False Alarms	2
Unsuccessful Searches	0
Lifeboat Unable to Complete Service	0
Others Coped	0

To Merchant and Fishing Vessels	3
To Pleasure Craft	0
To People	0
To Other Types of Casualty	0
Property Saved Value	£107,500
Services by Lifeboat	3
Services with Air Cooperation	0
Services Wind Over Force Seven	1
Services in Darkness	0
Services with Doctor/Auxillary on Board	0
Services Crew Claimed Salvage	0
Lifeboat Hours at Sea	10.4
Crew – Man Hours at Sea	65.7

1982

All Services (including assemblies)	13
Crew Assemblies (no launch)	0
Lives Saved	4
Persons Landed	1
Persons Brought In	0
Services to Crafts Saved/Landed	7
Successful Services	8
Co-ordinated by Coastguard	0
Non RNLI Lives Lost	1
Persons Injured	0
Hoax/False Alarms	0
Unsuccessful Searches	1
Lifeboat Unable to Complete Service	0
Others Coped	4
To Merchant and Fishing Vessels	10
To Pleasure Craft	2
To People	1
To Other Types of Casualty	0
Property Saved Value	£507,500
Services by Lifeboat	13
Services with Air Cooperation	2
Services Wind Over Force Seven	2
Services in Darkness	9
Services with Doctor/Auxillary on Board	1
Services Crew Claimed Salvage	0
Lifeboat Hours at Sea	77.3
Crew – Man Hours at Sea	512.4

1983

All Services (including assemblies)	6
Crew Assemblies (no launch)	0
Lives Saved	0
Persons Landed	3
Persons Brought In	0
Services to Crafts Saved/Landed	2
Successful Services	2
Co-ordinated by Coastguard	0
Non RNLI Lives Lost	0
Persons Injured	0
Hoax/False Alarms	1
Unsuccessful Searches	0
Lifeboat Unable to Complete Service	0
Others Coped	3
To Merchant and Fishing Vessels	4
To Pleasure Craft	0
To People	1
To Other Types of Casualty	1
Property Saved Value	£400
Services by Lifeboat	6
Services with Air Cooperation	0
Services Wind Over Force Seven	0
Services in Darkness	2
Services with Doctor/Auxillary on Board	0
Services Crew Claimed Salvage	0
Lifeboat Hours at Sea	19.5
Crew – Man Hours at Sea	153.3

1984

All Services (including assemblies)	19
Crew Assemblies (no launch)	0
Lives Saved	14
Persons Landed	2
Persons Brought In	0
Services to Crafts Saved/Landed	5
Successful Services	15
Co-ordinated by Coastguard	0
Non RNLI Lives Lost	2
Persons Injured	0
Hoax/False Alarms	4
Unsuccessful Searches	3

Lifeboat Unable to Complete Service	0
Others Coped	1
To Merchant and Fishing Vessels	10
To Pleasure Craft	2
To People	4
To Other Types of Casualty	3
Property Saved Value	£465,000
Services by Lifeboat	19
Services with Air Cooperation	3
Services Wind Over Force Seven	2
Services in Darkness	10
Services with Doctor/Auxillary on Board	2
Services Crew Claimed Salvage	0
Lifeboat Hours at Sea	91.1
Crew – Man Hours at Sea	582.1

1985

All Services (including assemblies)	14
Crew Assemblies (no launch)	0
Lives Saved	3
Persons Landed	1
Persons Brought In	0
Services to Crafts Saved/Landed	2
Successful Services	7
Co-ordinated by Coastguard	0
Non RNLI Lives Lost	5
Persons Injured	0
Hoax/False Alarms	3
Unsuccessful Searches	0
Lifeboat Unable to Complete Service	0
Others Coped	4
To Merchant and Fishing Vessels	5
To Pleasure Craft	3
To People	1
To Other Types of Casualty	5
Property Saved Value	£50,500
Services by Lifeboat	14
Services with Air Cooperation	4
Services Wind Over Force Seven	2
Services in Darkness	10
Services with Doctor/Auxillary on Board	0
Services Crew Claimed Salvage	0

Lifeboat Hours at Sea	99
Crew – Man Hours at Sea	987.6

1986

All Services (including assemblies)	20
Crew Assemblies (no launch)	0
Lives Saved	14
Persons Landed	0
Persons Brought In	0
Services to Crafts Saved/Landed	9
Successful Services	16
Co-ordinated by Coastguard	0
Non RNLI Lives Lost	5
Persons Injured	0
Hoax/False Alarms	1
Unsuccessful Searches	1
Lifeboat Unable to Complete Service	0
Others Coped	3
To Merchant and Fishing Vessels	12
To Pleasure Craft	7
To People	0
To Other Types of Casualty	1
Property Saved Value	£357,500
Services by Lifeboat	20
Services with Air Cooperation	1
Services Wind Over Force Seven	6
Services in Darkness	10
Services with Doctor/Auxillary on Board	0
Services Crew Claimed Salvage	0
Lifeboat Hours at Sea	96.9
Crew – Man Hours at Sea	586.4

1987

All Services (including assemblies)	19
Crew Assemblies (no launch)	0
Lives Saved	9
Persons Landed	4
Persons Brought In	0
Services to Crafts Saved/Landed	4
Successful Services	14
Co-ordinated by Coastguard	0
Non RNLI Lives Lost	1

Persons Injured	0
Hoax/False Alarms	4
Unsuccessful Searches	1
Lifeboat Unable to Complete Service	0
Others Coped	4
To Merchant and Fishing Vessels	12
To Pleasure Craft	2
To People	2
To Other Types of Casualty	3
Property Saved Value	£410,000
Services by Lifeboat	19
Services with Air Cooperation	1
Services Wind Over Force Seven	2
Services in Darkness	8
Services with Doctor/Auxillary on Board	1
Services Crew Claimed Salvage	0
Lifeboat Hours at Sea	80.4
Crew – Man Hours at Sea	515.7

1988

All Services (including assemblies)	9
Crew Assemblies (no launch)	0
Lives Saved	6
Persons Landed	1
Persons Brought In	
Services to Crafts Saved/Landed	2
Successful Services	5
Co-ordinated by Coastguard	
Non RNLI Lives Lost	1
Persons Injured	0
Hoax/False Alarms	0
Unsuccessful Searches	1
Lifeboat Unable to Complete Service	0
Others Coped	3
To Merchant and Fishing Vessels	6
To Pleasure Craft	3
To People	0
To Other Types of Casualty	0
Property Saved Value	£67,500
Services by Lifeboat	9
Services with Air Cooperation	2
Services Wind Over Force Seven	2

Services in Darkness	6
Services with Doctor/Auxillary on Board	0
Services Crew Claimed Salvage	0
Lifeboat Hours at Sea	36.3
Crew – Man Hours at Sea	238.3

1989

All Services (including assemblies)	16
Crew Assemblies (no launch)	0
Lives Saved	2
Persons Landed	2
Persons Brought In	2
Services to Crafts Saved/Landed	1
Successful Services	8
Co-ordinated by Coastguard	1
Non RNLI Lives Lost	7
Persons Injured	1
Hoax/False Alarms	1
Unsuccessful Searches	2
Lifeboat Unable to Complete Service	0
Others Coped	3
To Merchant and Fishing Vessels	9
To Pleasure Craft	0
To People	3
To Other Types of Casualty	2
Property Saved Value	£57,500
Services by Lifeboat	16
Services with Air Cooperation	4
Services Wind Over Force Seven	4
Services in Darkness	5
Services with Doctor/Auxillary on Board	3
Services Crew Claimed Salvage	0
Lifeboat Hours at Sea	55.5
Crew – Man Hours at Sea	308.8

1990

All Services (including assemblies)	10
Crew Assemblies (no launch)	0
Lives Saved	0
Persons Landed	1
Persons Brought In	0
Services to Crafts Saved/Landed	2

Successful Services	3
Co-ordinated by Coastguard	0
Non RNLI Lives Lost	2
Persons Injured	0
Hoax/False Alarms	0
Unsuccessful Searches	1
Lifeboat Unable to Complete Service	0
Others Coped	6
To Merchant and Fishing Vessels	6
To Pleasure Craft	3
To People	0
To Other Types of Casualty	1
Property Saved Value	£52,500
Services by Lifeboat	10
Services with Air Cooperation	4
Services Wind Over Force Seven	4
Services in Darkness	7
Services with Doctor/Auxillary on Board	1
Services Crew Claimed Salvage	0
Lifeboat Hours at Sea	29.4
Crew – Man Hours at Sea	164.5

1991

All Services (including assemblies)	19
Crew Assemblies (no launch)	0
Lives Saved	4
Persons Landed	1
Persons Brought In	0
Services to Crafts Saved/Landed	9
Successful Services	13
Co-ordinated by Coastguard	0
Non RNLI Lives Lost	5
Persons Injured	0
Hoax/False Alarms	0
Unsuccessful Searches	0
Lifeboat Unable to Complete Service	0
Others Coped	6
To Merchant and Fishing Vessels	6
To Pleasure Craft	11
To People	0
To Other Types of Casualty	2
Property Saved Value	£407,500

Services by Lifeboat   19
Services with Air Cooperation   6
Services Wind Over Force Seven   6
Services in Darkness   13
Services with Doctor/Auxillary on Board   0
Services Crew Claimed Salvage   0
Lifeboat Hours at Sea   83.7
Crew – Man Hours at Sea   555.2

1992
All Services (including assemblies)   10
Crew Assemblies (no launch)   0
Lives Saved   3
Persons Landed   3
Persons Brought In   0
Services to Crafts Saved/Landed   5
Successful Services   13
Co-ordinated by Coastguard   0
Non RNLI Lives Lost   0
Persons Injured   0
Hoax/False Alarms   1
Unsuccessful Searches   0
Lifeboat Unable to Complete Service   0
Others Coped   4
To Merchant and Fishing Vessels   4
To Pleasure Craft   5
To People   0
To Other Types of Casualty   1
Property Saved Value   £453,000
Services by Lifeboat   10
Services with Air Cooperation   3
Services Wind Over Force Seven   0
Services in Darkness   3
Services with Doctor/Auxillary on Board   0
Services Crew Claimed Salvage   0
Lifeboat Hours at Sea   25.1
Crew – Man Hours at Sea   165.8

1993
All Services (including assemblies)   25
Crew Assemblies (no launch)   0

Lives Saved	16
Persons Landed	1
Persons Brought In	11
Services to Crafts Saved/Landed	5
Successful Services	13
Co-ordinated by Coastguard	2
Non RNLI Lives Lost	0
Persons Injured	0
Hoax/False Alarms	5
Unsuccessful Searches	1
Lifeboat Unable to Complete Service	0
Others Coped	6
To Merchant and Fishing Vessels	4
To Pleasure Craft	5
To People	0
To Other Types of Casualty	1
Property Saved Value	£1,007,500
Services by Lifeboat	25
Services with Air Cooperation	3
Services Wind Over Force Seven	8
Services in Darkness	15
Services with Doctor/Auxillary on Board	0
Services Crew Claimed Salvage	0
Lifeboat Hours at Sea	101.2
Crew – Man Hours at Sea	657.8

1994

All Services (including assemblies)	14
Crew Assemblies (no launch)	0
Lives Saved	13
Persons Landed	2
Persons Brought In	5
Services to Crafts Saved/Landed	5
Successful Services	12
Co-ordinated by Coastguard	14
Non RNLI Lives Lost	4
Persons Injured	2
Hoax/False Alarms	0
Unsuccessful Searches	0
Lifboat Unable to Complete Service	0
Others Coped	2
To Merchant and Fishing Vessels	9

To Pleasure Craft	4
To People	1
To Other Types of Casualty	0
Property Saved Value	£453,000
Services by Lifeboat	14
Services with Air Cooperation	3
Services Wind Over Force Seven	3
Services in Darkness	12
Services with Doctor/Auxillary on Board	1
Services Crew Claimed Salvage	0
Lifeboat Hours at Sea	52.2
Crew – Man Hours at Sea	323.6

1995

All Services (including assemblies)	19
Crew Assemblies (no launch)	1
Lives Saved	9
Persons Landed	5
Persons Brought In	30
Services to Crafts Saved/Landed	7
Successful Services	11
Co-ordinated by Coastguard	18
Non RNLI Lives Lost	1
Persons Injured	0
Hoax/False Alarms	3
Unsuccessful Searches	0
Lifeboat Unable to Complete Service	0
Others Coped	4
To Merchant and Fishing Vessels	11
To Pleasure Craft	3
To People	2
To Other Types of Casualty	3
Property Saved Value	£688,000
Services by Lifeboat	19
Services with Air Cooperation	5
Services Wind Over Force Seven	2
Services in Darkness	12
Services with Doctor/Auxillary on Board	0
Services Crew Claimed Salvage	0
Lifeboat Hours at Sea	60.8
Crew – Man Hours at Sea	366.6

1996

All Services (including assemblies)	27
Crew Assemblies (no launch)	0
Lives Saved	10
Persons Landed	14
Persons Brought In	28
Services to Crafts Saved/Landed	14
Successful Services	21
Co-ordinated by Coastguard	0
Non RNLI Lives Lost	2
Persons Injured	1
Hoax/False Alarms	2
Unsuccessful Searches	1
Lifeboat Unable to Complete Service	0
Others Coped	3
To Merchant and Fishing Vessels	20
To Pleasure Craft	6
To People	1
To Other Types of Casualty	0
Property Saved Value	£1,300,000
Services by Lifeboat	27
Services with Air Cooperation	3
Services Wind Over Force Seven	6
Services in Darkness	14
Services with Doctor/Auxillary on Board	0
Services Crew Claimed Salvage	0
Lifeboat Hours at Sea	117.4
Crew – Man Hours at Sea	790.8

1997

All Services (including assemblies)	32
Crew Assemblies (no launch)	0
Lives Saved	9
Persons Landed	6
Persons Brought In	23
Services to Crafts Saved/Landed	9
Successful Services	17
Co-ordinated by Coastguard	0
Non RNLI Lives Lost	4
Persons Injured	2
Hoax/False Alarms	1
Unsuccessful Searches	8

Lifeboat Unable to Complete Service	0
Others Coped	6
To Merchant and Fishing Vessels	15
To Pleasure Craft	6
To People	11
To Other Types of Casualty	0
Property Saved Value	£229,050
Services by Lifeboat	32
Services with Air Cooperation	6
Services Wind Over Force Seven	1
Services in Darkness	14
Services with Doctor/Auxillary on Board	0
Services Crew Claimed Salvage	0
Lifeboat Hours at Sea	106
Crew – Man Hours at Sea	716.6

1998

All Services (including assemblies)	23
Crew Assemblies (no launch)	0
Lives Saved	22
Persons Landed	10
Persons Brought In	32
Services to Crafts Saved/Landed	11
Successful Services	16
Co-ordinated by Coastguard	0
Non RNLI Lives Lost	0
Persons Injured	0
Hoax/False Alarms	1
Unsuccessful Searches	0
Lifeboat Unable to Complete Service	0
Others Coped	6
To Merchant and Fishing Vessels	14
To Pleasure Craft	7
To People	1
To Other Types of Casualty	1
Property Saved Value	£1,170,000
Services by Lifeboat	23
Services with Air Cooperation	4
Services Wind Over Force Seven	0
Services in Darkness	10
Services with Doctor/Auxillary on Board	0
Services Crew Claimed Salvage	0

Lifeboat Hours at Sea	61.1
Crew – Man Hours at Sea	399.8

1999

All Services (including assemblies)	16
Crew Assemblies (no launch)	0
Lives Saved	5
Persons Landed	2
Persons Brought In	10
Services to Crafts Saved/Landed	4
Successful Services	8
Co-ordinated by Coastguard	0
Non RNLI Lives Lost	0
Persons Injured	1
Hoax/False Alarms	4
Unsuccessful Searches	0
Lifeboat Unable to Complete Service	0
Others Coped	4
To Merchant and Fishing Vessels	9
To Pleasure Craft	1
To People	2
To Other Types of Casualty	4
Property Saved Value	£600,000
Services by Lifeboat	16
Services with Air Cooperation	6
Services Wind Over Force Seven	4
Services in Darkness	9
Services with Doctor/Auxillary on Board	0
Services Crew Claimed Salvage	0
Lifeboat Hours at Sea	53.1
Crew – Man Hours at Sea	357.6

2000

All Services (including assemblies)	25
Crew Assemblies (no launch)	0
Lives Saved	1
Persons Landed	17
Persons Brought In	23
Services to Crafts Saved/Landed	10
Successful Services	18
Co-ordinated by Coastguard	0
Non RNLI Lives Lost	0

Persons Injured	1
Hoax/False Alarms	3
Unsuccessful Searches	1
Lifeboat Unable to Complete Service	0
Others Coped	3
To Merchant and Fishing Vessels	13
To Pleasure Craft	6
To People	3
To Other Types of Casualty	3
Property Saved Value	£1,748,000
Services by Lifeboat	25
Services with Air Cooperation	3
Services Wind Over Force Seven	5
Services in Darkness	10
Services with Doctor/Auxillary on Board	0
Services Crew Claimed Salvage	0
Lifeboat Hours at Sea	71.1
Crew – Man Hours at Sea	443.9

2001

All Services (including assemblies)	13
Crew Assemblies (no launch)	0
Lives Saved	0
Persons Landed	15
Persons Brought In	12
Services to Crafts Saved/Landed	3
Successful Services	8
Co-ordinated by Coastguard	0
Non RNLI Lives Lost	0
Persons Injured	3
Hoax/False Alarms	3
Unsuccessful Searches	1
Lifeboat Unable to Complete Service	0
Others Coped	1
To Merchant and Fishing Vessels	9
To Pleasure Craft	1
To People	2
To Other Types of Casualty	1
Property Saved Value	£138,000
Services by Lifeboat	13
Services with Air Cooperation	2
Services Wind Over Force Seven	1

Services in Darkness	6
Services with Doctor/Auxillary on Board	0
Services Crew Claimed Salvage	0
Lifeboat Hours at Sea	37
Crew – Man Hours at Sea	238.5

2002

All Services (including assemblies)	25
Crew Assemblies (no launch)	0
Lives Saved	6
Persons Landed	21
Persons Brought In	24
Services to Crafts Saved/Landed	10
Successful Services	17
Co-ordinated by Coastguard	0
Non RNLI Lives Lost	2
Persons Injured	0
Hoax/False Alarms	4
Unsuccessful Searches	1
Lifeboat Unable to Complete Service	0
Others Coped	3
To Merchant and Fishing Vessels	12
To Pleasure Craft	8
To People	4
To Other Types of Casualty	1
Property Saved Value	£332,700
Services by Lifeboat	25
Services with Air Cooperation	5
Services Wind Over Force Seven	5
Services in Darkness	12
Services with Doctor/Auxillary on Board	0
Services Crew Claimed Salvage	0
Lifeboat Hours at Sea	76.1
Crew – Man Hours at Sea	543.3

2003

All Services (including assemblies)	17
Crew Assemblies (no launch)	0
Lives Saved	0
Persons Landed	16
Persons Brought In	33
Services to Crafts Saved/Landed	11

Successful Services	14
Co-ordinated by Coastguard	0
Non RNLI Lives Lost	1
Persons Injured	0
Hoax/False Alarms	2
Unsuccessful Searches	0
Lifeboat Unable to Complete Service	0
Others Coped	1
To Merchant and Fishing Vessels	5
To Pleasure Craft	8
To People	2
To Other Types of Casualty	2
Property Saved Value	£2,235,235
Services by Lifeboat	17
Services with Air Cooperation	1
Services Wind Over Force Seven	3
Services in Darkness	14
Services with Doctor/Auxillary on Board	0
Services Crew Claimed Salvage	0
Lifeboat Hours at Sea	37
Crew – Man Hours at Sea	248.6

2004

All Services (including assemblies)	23
Crew Assemblies (no launch)	0
Lives Saved	0
Persons Landed	4
Persons Brought In	41
Services to Crafts Saved/Landed	14
Successful Services	20
Co-ordinated by Coastguard	0
Non RNLI Lives Lost	1
Persons Injured	0
Hoax/False Alarms	1
Unsuccessful Searches	0
Lifeboat Unable to Complete Service	0
Others Coped	2
To Merchant and Fishing Vessels	15
To Pleasure Craft	6
To People	2
To Other Types of Casualty	0
Property Saved Value	£2,235,235

Services by Lifeboat	23
Services with Air Cooperation	4
Services Wind Over Force Seven	1
Services in Darkness	8
Services with Doctor/Auxillary on Board	1
Services Crew Claimed Salvage	0
Lifeboat Hours at Sea	42.7
Crew – Man Hours at Sea	255.4

2005

All Services (including assemblies)	19
Crew Assemblies (no launch)	0
Lives Saved	0
Persons Landed	3
Persons Brought In	50
Services to Crafts Saved/Landed	13
Successful Services	15
Co-ordinated by Coastguard	0
Non RNLI Lives Lost	0
Persons Injured	0
Hoax/False Alarms	3
Unsuccessful Searches	0
Lifeboat Unable to Complete Service	0
Others Coped	1
To Merchant and Fishing Vessels	10
To Pleasure Craft	5
To People	1
To Other Types of Casualty	3
Property Saved Value	£599,037
Services by Lifeboat	19
Services with Air Cooperation	0
Services Wind Over Force Seven	0
Services in Darkness	8
Services with Doctor/Auxillary on Board	0
Services Crew Claimed Salvage	0
Lifeboat Hours at Sea	45.4
Crew – Man Hours at Sea	288.7

2006

All Services (including assemblies)	19
Crew Assemblies (no launch)	0
Lives Saved	0

Persons Landed	0
Persons Brought In	21
Services to Crafts Saved/Landed	13
Successful Services	8
Co-ordinated by Coastguard	0
Non RNLI Lives Lost	2
Persons Injured	0
Hoax/False Alarms	0
Unsuccessful Searches	3
Lifeboat Unable to Complete Service	0
Others Coped	3
To Merchant and Fishing Vessels	7
To Pleasure Craft	5
To People	2
To Other Types of Casualty	5
Property Saved Value	£149,000
Services by Lifeboat	19
Services with Air Cooperation	0
Services Wind Over Force Seven	1
Services in Darkness	3
Services with Doctor/Auxillary on Board	0
Services Crew Claimed Salvage	0
Lifeboat Hours at Sea	42.1
Crew – Man Hours at Sea	258.7

2007

All Services (including assemblies)	25
Crew Assemblies (no launch)	0
Lives Saved	0
Persons Landed	0
Persons Brought In	28
Services to Crafts Saved/Landed	15
Successful Services	15
Co-ordinated by Coastguard	25
Non RNLI Lives Lost	1
Persons Injured	0
Hoax/False Alarms	2
Unsuccessful Searches	3
Lifeboat Unable to Complete Service	0
Others Coped	5
To Merchant and Fishing Vessels	10
To Pleasure Craft	7

To People	4
To Other Types of Casualty	4
Property Saved Value	£885,000
Services by Lifeboat	25
Services with Air Cooperation	0
Services Wind Over Force Seven	5
Services in Darkness	4
Services with Doctor/Auxillary on Board	0
Services Crew Claimed Salvage	0
Lifeboat Hours at Sea	71.1
Crew – Man Hours at Sea	428.7

2008

All Services (including assemblies)	23
Crew Assemblies (no launch)	0
Lives Saved	5
Persons Landed	1
Persons Brought In	38
Services to Crafts Saved/Landed	10
Successful Services	16
Co-ordinated by Coastguard	23
Non RNLI Lives Lost	0
Persons Injured	0
Hoax/False Alarms	4
Unsuccessful Searches	1
Lifeboat Unable to Complete Service	0
Others Coped	2
To Merchant and Fishing Vessels	5
To Pleasure Craft	11
To People	4
To Other Types of Casualty	0
Property Saved Value	32,044,000
Services by Lifeboat	23
Services with Air Cooperation	0
Services Wind Over Force Seven	4
Services in Darkness	3
Services with Doctor/Auxillary on Board	0
Services Crew Claimed Salvage	0
Lifeboat Hours at Sea	66.10
Crew – Man Hours at Sea	397

APPENDIX 5

Valentia Lifeboat Station – Boat Record

ON	Name	Term	Launches	Lives Saved	Cost
	Mary	1864–80	6	Nil	£223 6s
	Crosby Leonard	1880–90	Nil	Nil	£303
174	as above	1890–6	4	Nil	£352
690	*C&S*	1946–7	2	Nil	£8,424
687	*BASP*	1947–51	14	2	£7,519
717	*AED*	1951–7	57	80	£10,119
938	*Rowland Watts*	1957–83	158	132	£33,500
1082	*Margaret Frances Love*	1983–96	192	73	£376,00
1218	*John and Margaret Doig*	1996–present			£1,580,000

The names of all lifeboats are preceded by the letters ' R.N.L.B.' O.N. 687 was not formally assigned to Valentia but given the length of time she was on temporary station duty is included above for the sake of continuity.

Lifeboats which did Temporary Duty at Valentia.

ON	Name	Original Station
709	*City of Bradford 1*	Humber
733	*Mary Stanford*	Ballycotton
755	*Peter and Sarah Blake*	Fenit
700	*KECF*	Rosslare harbour
802	*City of Edinburgh*	Wick
718	*William and Harriett*	Stornoway
898	*Joseph Hiram Chadwick*	Padstow
923	*John Galletly Hyndeman*	Stronsay

912	*Euphrosyne Kendal*	St Peter Port, Guernsey
1067	*Hyman Winstone*	Holyhead
1108	*Margaret Russell Frazer*	Built for Relief Fleet
1150	*Hibernia*	Built for Relief Fleet
1254	*Volunteer Spirit*	Built for Relief Fleet

APPENDIX 6

The Ancillary Services

The Lighthouses and Coastguard
Coast Lifesaving Service

The Lighthouses

No vessel or lifeboat can operate without lighthouses. The Principal Lighthouses in the bailiewick of the Valentia lifeboat are Loop Head, Inistearaght, Cromwell Point, Valentia Island, Valentia Leading Lights, Skellig Rock, Bull Rock and Mizen Head. The lighthouse men, keeping a voluntary watch, have over the years been instrumental in saving many lives. All the offshore lighthouses have become automated. A computer can keep the light flashing and switch on an emergency generator. Unfortunately it can't see a flare and report it. The lives of seafarers run an extra risk thanks to automation. That's progress.

Loop Head 52.34 North 9.56 West

The first lighthouse on Loop Head was one of four known Irish stone-vaulted cottage-type lighthouses built in about 1670. These cottages accommodated the light keeper and his family in two or three rooms and had an internal stone stairway between two of the rooms leading up to a platform on the roof where a coal burning brazier or chauffer was positioned. Part of the old cottage with its battered outside wall can still be seen near the light keepers' dwellings.

The light seems to have fallen into disuse towards the end of the seventeenth century because it was re-established in 1720. This followed the petitioning of the Irish Parliament in 1717 for a light on the Head by the Aldermen and Merchants of Limerick. In 1802, the cottage-lighthouse was replaced by a more conventional lighthouse and the era of the coal fire light was ended.

The lighthouse was built by Thomas Rogers, who was also the contractor. The tower was roughly the same height as the present one – 23m overall with the lantern 84m (277 feet) above high water, and had four rooms and a lantern. The ground-floor room was an oilstore and access to the first floor or entrance room was by an internal staircase of nineteen steps. An internal spiral staircase connected the other two rooms and the lantern.

The 12 foot diameter lantern contained twelve oil lamps, each with its own concave parabolic reflector. The reflected light shone through a twenty-two-inch diameter convex lense of solid glass, not unlike the 'Bottle Glass' or 'Bulls Eye' into windows of modern Pseudo-Georgian Houses.

By 1811 the light keeper was living in an adjoining cottage and not in the tower. The number of lamps and reflectors in the lantern had been increased by fifteen by 1825. During 1836 the Limerick Chamber of Commerce complained of the poor light and went as far as suggesting that the tower should be rebuilt. The inspector investigated the complaint and reported back to the board that the light was as good as most lights around the coast and did not warrant immediate attention. However, seven years later, towards the end of 1843, he did propose that a new tower and optic be provided.

The Ballast Board agreed and by June 1844 the seal was attached to the contract for Mr William Burgess of Limerick to build a new tower, approximately 30 feet from the 1802 tower in an east-north-east direction. The new tower, designed by the inspector, George Halpin, was completed early in 1854 and took over from the 1802 tower on 1 May that year. In order not to obstruct the light from the new tower, the old one, of almost identical height had to be demolished in daylight hours prior to 1 May. The light was altered on a number of occasions with a new intermittent light coming into operation in March 1969. An explosive fog signal was established in 1898. This remained in operation until 1972 when it was discontinued. The light itself was improved in 1912 and was converted to electric from vapourising paraffin in 1971

During 1955 a radio beacon was established, transmitting the morse signal L.P. (. -. . - -) every two minutes during fog. This was changed to continual transmission irrespective of weather in May 1964 and on 9 December 1977 Loophead's Radio Beacon was grouped with the new beacon at Slyne Head Marine VHF and SSB Radio was also provided at the station.

Inistearaght 52.04 North 10.40 West

This is the most westerly of the Blasket group of islands. The lighthouse, with two keepers and their families, was established on 1 May 1879. The light is 84 metres above high water and its character is two flashes every twenty seconds. It was converted to vapourised paraffin in 1909 and to electric in 1961 with a candle power of 1.4 million. A diaphone fog signal, established in 1925 was replaced by an electric horn in 1980. Like Skelligs, the keepers and their families were housed by 1900 in shore dwellings at Valentia from where boat reliefs were made. When the dwellings were sold in 1964 the reliefs were carried out from Castletownbere and by October 1968 a helicopter had taken over. Now this light is unmanned.

Cromwellpoint, Valentia Island 51.56 North 10.19 West

This is a light to guide vessels from sea safely through the northern entrance to Valentia harbour and guide them past Harbour Rock. Maurice Fitzgerald, Knight of Kerry, applied for a light in 1828. The board deferred the matter and in 1837 the board was again referred to the matter by Maurice O'Connell, Esq. On inspection of the area, Mr G. Halpin recommended that a light be placed at the point. Sanction from Trinity House came in April 1837 and the tower was built by the board's workmen to the design of George Halpin Senior. The cut stone tower, painted white is 54 feet above high water and could be seen for 12 miles in clear weather. The old walls of one of Cromwell's two forts (the other was at Sculgaphort opposite Portmagee, both being built in 1653) were mostly retained with only minimum necessary alterations being made. While the light shone from 1 February 1841 the establishment was not completed fully until the end of 1842 and the total cost was £10,846 17s. The station went unmanned on 4 November 1947 and the light was altered to flashing red with a white sector clear of Harbour Rock. In 1966, on 8 July the light went electric and the white light candlepower increased to 34,500. A stand-by generator comes into operation in the event of a mains power failure.

Valentia Leading Lights

Two unlit beacons beside and on the north side of the Glanleam Road, 25 and 43 metres above high water, were established on 20 January 1981 to give daylight guidance to vessels past Harbour Rock, locally called 'The Perch'. The rock has a 12 metre high pole painted yellow and black with East Cones. The beacons were lit on 1 May 1913. Whilst unwatched, keepers ashore from Skelligs or Tearaght saw to them. The front light was converted to electricity on 16 August 1967; the rear light was discontinued, but was re-established on 9 March 1977.

Skellig Rock Lighthouse 51.46 North 10.32 West

'The Skelligs' are known worldwide as a bird sanctuary and monastic ruin. The existence of a lighthouse there, if noticed, is rarely recognised for the feat of engineering that it is.

Sir Maurice Fitzgerald first sought a lighthouse on Skellig Micheal. Fitzgerald, Knight of Kerry, received approval in 1820. The Corporation for Improving the Port of Dublin – predecessors of today's Commissioners of Irish Lights – paid the princely sum of £800 to Butler of Waterville for the island.

To Engineer George Halpin fell the hapless task of building not one, but two lighthouses on this barren isolated stalk of bleak rock. It was felt necessary to build two so that Skellig could be distinguished from Loop Head to the north and Cape Clear to the south. That this 111-mile stretch of the most fearsome and dangerous coast in the world remained unlit for so long is a total mystery.

One light was to be above Seal Cove 175 feet above sea level and the other at the western extremity 372 feet above sea level.

The lighthouses were 780 feet apart with the towers painted white. A principal and an assistant keeper together with their families were attached to each station. In addition to the lighthouses themselves, 3,200 feet of approach road had to be built from the landing place at Blind Man's Cove. When the Inistearaght light to the north was lit the upper lighthouse was discontinued. As with Tearaght, the Skellig personnel were housed at Valentia by 1900 and 'the relief' became quite a local event with the vessels like the *Nabro*, the *Lerne*, the *Isolda*, the *Valonia* and the *Granuaile* being regular visitors to the harbour. The light was improved in 1909 and a fog signal was in operation from 1914 until 1953. On 25 May 1967 the light was converted to electric and the dwellings were modernised. Relief by helicopter commenced in 1968 and the light went automatic in the latter part of 1987.

Bull Rock 51.35 North 10.18 West

A lighthouse established on the Calf Rock on 30 June 1966 marked the group of islands. The Bull, Cow, Calf and Heifer off the south-west corner of Dursey Island and the entrance to Bantry Bay. The tower was of cast iron and was 42 metres above high water.

On 27 November 1881 a great storm swept all but the lower room into the sea. A temporary light was established on Dursey Island until the light on the Bull Rock came into operation on 1 January 1889. An explosive fog signal established in 1889 was changed to a triple siren in 1902. Due to their remoteness, dwellings on Dursey were abandoned by the keepers in 1940 and sold in 1946.

Mizenhead. 51.27 North 9.49 West

The lifeboat service does not have hard and fast boundaries. Mizen Head would normally be the southernmost point on Valentia lifeboat's 'patch', though they did go 75 miles south-west of it on a mammoth service to the *George X* on 1 October 1971.

The Board of Trade gave sanction for a lighthouse to be erected at Mizen Head on the 28 April 1905. The lighthouse conference in April 1906 agreed that only a fog signal was necessary at Mizen and the new station would be put in the care of the principal keeper at the Fastnet. On 18 October 1907 sanction was given for Thorne and Co. to build a new reinforced concrete bridge at a cost of £1,200. Following the wreck of the SS *Trada* at Mizen on 22 December 1908, when sixty-three lives were saved by the resident engineer and the workmen, the lack of a fog signal was blamed. The master of the vessel so informed the enquiry which was held on 26 January 1909. The fog signal was established on 3 May 1909.

In July 1909, the keeper's dwellings were whitewashed to make a better day mark. On 20 May 1920, the station was raided by armed men and all the explosives taken away. All fog signal stations using explosives around the coast were closed as the Government would not give them protection. The signal was re-established on 29 February 1924. A lighthouse was established on the Mizen on 1 October 1959 and is of 4,600 candle power, visible for 13 miles in clear weather. The staff at Mizen were commended by the board on 2 February 1940 for help given by them, and local people, to the twelve rescued crew members of the Norwegian trawler *Songa* which had been sunk by a German submarine.

On 29 September 1985 the yacht *Taurima* struck the Mizen. Principal Keeper Richard Foran was lowered on a rope down the cliff face and using a flashlamp kept the survivors advised of how to avoid rocks which would reef and sink their inflatable rubber dingy and life-raft. Assistant Keeper Michael Knessey and Richard Cummins, acting assistant keeper, kept Foran informed of the progress of the two lifeboats racing to the scene. Valentia and Baltimore lifeboats were both alerted and launched. At 4.03 a.m. the survivors were aboard the *Charles Henry* from Baltimore and the *Margaret Frances Love* returned to station. It was not until the journey home was under way that one of the Baltimore Crew realised that one of the survivors was Mr Charles J. Haughey TD, then leader of the opposition in Dáil Eireann. His comment 'Jayzas, is it yourself? This isn't a rescue, this is a catch', is likely to remain on record for some considerable time.

Coastguard Coast Lifesaving Service

There is a unit of the Coast Lifesaving Service at Knightstown and it is locally referred to as 'The Rocket Car' and the name is apt. It carries rope ladders and a tripod and rockets and a breeches buoy. That a horse cart was still the method of transportation provided certainly caused some great mirth to visitors who watched an exercise in August 1985. The formation of the Irish Marine Emergency Service, now named the Irish Coastguard, transformed this service.

Circumstances can arise where rescue can only be effected from the shore. A breeches buoy is effectively a round lifebelt with a canvas trousers or breeches attached. The lifeboat also carries one of these. Operated from the shore, a rocket is fired over the casualty and carries a messenger, or light rope. On to this is attached the main rope, a three-inch hawser which is secured on board the casualty. The other end of the hawser is passed through a pulley on top of a tripod ashore and secured to a luff, which is itself secured to a stake holdfast. The breeches buoy itself hangs by a travelling block (pulley) from the hawser. Attached to the block are two whip lines, one end passing through a block secured on board the casualty. The other line runs from the shore side of the breeches buoy to the shore, this is the lee whip, the other the weather whip. The whips are used to pull the buoy back and forth from the ship. The whips are operated from boxes kept well apart to prevent the lines being swept across the buoy and throwing the occupant out, or to prevent them fouling each other.

In Valentia there is some hazy recollection of one assembly for a vessel with faulty steering off the Wireless Point, prior to the *Big Cat* episode. The sea is totally unpredictable and it is a fool who would state that the Coast Lifesaving Unit is superfluous because there is not a bit statistical list of rescues on file. It must be remembered also that in recent years the Shannon Estuary has brought massive shipping to this coast. Within weeks of the rescue the Coast Lifesaving Unit at Valentia received new equipment. The old transport – a horse cart which the British Coastguard had left when leaving – has been donated to and is an exhibit at the local Heritage Centre in Knightstown where it joins the history of the Lifeboat, Radio Station, Cable Station, Slate Quarry and sundry other displays of former times on the historic island of Valentia.

The people of Valentia had united to meet the challenge of the sea in the best traditions of seafaring people and their courage, self sacrifice and hospitality were justly commended by the Minister for the Marine Mr Brendan Daly and by the media. Following the nine-hour service in savage conditions. Coxswain Seanie Murphy received a framed letter of thanks from the Chairman of the RNLI for his seamanship and leadership. Mechanic Joseph Houlihan, Assistant Mechanic James Murphy and crew members John Sheehan received letters of thanks from the Chief of Operations. The director wrote letters to the members of the Coast Lifesaving Unit. The skill of the coxswain in co-ordinating the rescue was commented on and highly praised by all concerned.

APPENDIX 7

The Flank Stations

Fenit Lifeboat Station

From 1879 to 1946, Fenit station had provided lifeboat cover for most of the Kerry Coast, until Valentia re-opened in 1946. The Fenit station was closed in April 1969 after eight-eight launches and fifty-six lives saved. The lifeboats which served there were *Admiral Butcher*, 1879-90; *Louise & Emma*, 1890-5; *John Willmot*, 1895-1923; *James Stephens No. 20*, 1923-8; *John A. Hay*, 1928-32 (this was the first lifeboat built as a motor lifeboat); *Peter and Sarah Blake*, 1932-58; *Hilton Briggs*, 1958-69. Fenit station re-opened in 1994. The station now operates a Trent class lifeboat ON 1238 (14-27) Robert Hwyel Jones Williams and also a 'D' class inflatable D-726 Bradley and Sonia. Fenit is currently the Northern Flank Station.

Castletownbere Lifeboat Station

Castletownbere Lifeboat Station was opened in 1997. The lifeboat *Roy & Barbara Harding* (ON 1118) 52-36 arrived at Castletown on 25 October 1997. Following the usual period of evaluation the station was formally established on 7 April 1998. The station currently operates a Severn class lifeboat ON 1277 (17-44) RNLB *Annette Hutton*.

There is a peculiar but interesting coincidence here. The Hutton Family were major coach builders in Dublin. When Queen Victoria visited Ireland she ordered a 'Hutton' coach for 'The Palace'.

In 2004 when the Lifeboat College in Poole was opened by Queen Elizabeth II she was taken for a trip in Poole harbour on board the Castletownbere Lifeboat. The crew were there to do their training and collect their new lifeboat.

During the time that Fenit was closed and before Castletownbere opened the flank stations were at Baltimore and Galway Bay. This is now named Aran Islands Lifeboat Station.

Baltimore

Baltimore Station was approved in 1913. Due to the war it did not open until 1919. The boathouse which was erected at Bull Point is still in use today. It is anticipated that it will house the Inshore lifeboat when a Tamar class comes on station. The Tamar will operate from a pen. The lifeboats which served there were:

The Duke of Connaught, re-named *Shamrock* in 1920 (ON 649) on station until 1950 with 43 launches and 34 lives saved.
Sarah Tilson (ON 854) 1950 to 1978 with 70 launches and 21 lives saved.
The *Robert* (ON 955) 1978 to 1984 with 44 launches and 31 lives saved.
Charles Henry (ON 1015) 1984 to 1987 with 35 launches 28 lives saved
Ethel Mary (ON 949) 1987 to 1988 with 11 launches and 5 lives saved.
The Current Tyne class lifeboat ON 1137 *Hilda Jarrett* had been on station since March 1987.
This station also operates an Atlantic class lifeboat B 708 *Bessie*.

Galway Bay

Galway Bay Lifeboat Station was opened at Kilronan on the Aran Islands in 1927. The lifeboats that served there were:

William Evans (ON 653) 1927 to 1939 launched 24 times and saved 29 lives.
KECF (ON 700) 1939 to 1952 launched 37 times and saved 48 lives.
(ON 700 was the first lifeboat to be fitted with wireless. On 24 June 1927 while stationed at Rosslare harbour she saved the crew of the lugger *Mona* the first service by an RNLI lifeboats so equipped.)
Mabel Marion Thompson (ON 818) 1952 to 1968 launched 177 times and saved 72 lives.
Joseph Hiram Chadwick (ON 898) 1968 to 1977 launched 198 times and saved 7 lives.
Frank Spillar Locke (ON 939) 1977 to 1985 launched 130 times and saved 7 lives.
R. Hope Roberts (ON 1011) 1985 to 1987 launched 37 times and saved 5 lives.
Roy and Barbara Harding (ON 1118) 1987 to 1997 Launched 315 times and saved 43 lives.

The station was renamed Aran Islands Lifeboat Station from 1 August 1995. (This was to avoid confusion when a station was opened at Galway City).

The lifeboat on station since 1997 is the David Kirkaldy (ON 1217). A Severn class lifeboat (17-06).

APPENDIX 8

RNLB *BASP*

There is a Lifeboat Museum at Chatham Dockyard. Here various lifeboats are being preserved. One boat which served at Valentia is included in the restoration and preservation programme. Accordingly, it is fitting to record her details and service as for the foreseeable future she is the only lifeboat to have served at Valentia which will be preserved.

Built in 1924 by J. Samuel White & Co. at Cowes, Isle of Wight. Forty-five foot Watson class lifeboat as already described. Cost £7,519. Station: Yarmouth, Isle of Wight.

Date	Casualty	Result
11/11/1925	Schooner *Flying Foam* of Bridgewater	Saved boat and rescued 5
15/02/1926	SS *Urkiloa Mendi* of Bilboa	Stood by
15/04/1926	SS *Haslemere* of Southampton	Saved 5
25/04/1926	Yacht *Alektor* of Shoreham	Saved boat and rescued 3
24/03/1927	SS *Yapalaga* of Philadelphia	Landed an injured man
25/03/1927	Schooner *Annemarie* of Hamburg	Took out doctor
26/06/1927	Ketch *Nelly*	Stood by
30/07/1927	Paddle steamer *Queen* of Southampton	stood by
12/08/1927	Sailing boat *Jean* of Yarmouth	Saved boat rescued 4
23/04/1928	Admiralty drifter *Cold Snap*	Gave help
24/08/1931	Yacht *Patience*	gave help
17/01/1931	Speed boat *Hoity Toity* of Christchurch	Saved boat rescued 1
15/05/1932	SS *Roumelian* of Liverpool	Landed 4

17/07/1932	Yacht *Daedelus* of Cowes	Saved boat and rescued 1
28/08/1934	Motor launch *Oreron* of Totland Bay	Saved boat and rescued 6
04/09/1934	Sailing boat *Vigilant* of Totland Bay	Saved boat and rescued 2
25/10/1934	Yacht *Casita* of Penzance	Saved yacht and rescued 3

Falmouth Station 1934 – 1940

Date	Casualty	Result
24/12/1935	SS *Brightside* of Liverpool	Helped to moor vessel
01/06/1938	Yacht *Salonique* of St Mawes	Search failed
01/06/1938	Yacht *Tender*	Saved dinghy and rescued 3
05/08/1938	SS *Esther Maria* of Esjberg	Assisted to refloat vessel
05/10/1938	MV *Redhead* of London	Landed 4
02/11/1939	SS *Pink Rose* of Liverpool	Escorted ship to harbour

Valentia Island Station 1947 - 1951

Date	Casualty	Result
26/06/1949	Rowing boat	Gave help
22/02/1950	FV *Pride* of Ballinskelligs	Saved boat & rescued 2
24/03/1950	Relieved Skelligs Rock Lighthouse	
26/03/1950	Relieved Inistearaght Lighthhouse	
01/08/1950	FV *Ocean Star* of Dingle	Escorted boat

The lifeboat launched nine other times from Valentia when they could find no ships in distress, were not wanted, or could do nothing. During her service career and including all stations where she served as Station Boat or in a reserve capacity the *BASP* launched on service a total of eight-one times and saved a total of thirty-seven lives. She was sold out of service in 1955.

APPENDIX 9

Lifeboat Crew List

(This list has been compiled from various sources. Some records were illegible. It is as accurate as possible from the sources available. Any omissions are regretted.)

B
Barry, William (Bill) (fleet mechanic)
Bartlett, Charlie
Breslin, Frank
Burke, D.

C
Cahill, Joanne
Cahill, T.
Casey, J.
Casey Sean
Condon, J.
Connell, T.
Connolly, J.
Connolly, Martin
Connolly Richard
Cotter, Paddy (fleet mechanic)
Curran, James
Curran, John
Curran, J.F.
Curran, John J.
Curran, Michael
Curran, Noel
Curtin, Brendan

Curtin, John
Curtin, Pat

D
Daly, Denis
Daly, T.
Devane, Kevin
Dore, John (mechanic)
Donovan, N.

F
Flanagan, James (fleet mechanic)
Fitzgerald, W (fleet mechanic)
Foran, Leo
Foran, M.

G
Gallagher, D.
Gallagher, John
Gallagher, P.
Galvin, Jim
Gannon, Mark (fleet mechanic)
Gilligan, Tommy
Grandfield, Liam
Grandfield, Patrick

H
Hall, A.
Harty, P.
Hillier, Syd
Houlihan, Joseph (mechanic) (Bronze Medal)
Houlihan, Leo (mechanic)
Houlihan, Pat
Houlihan, Peadar

L
Lavelle, Desmond (second cox)
Linnane, Adrian
Lynch, James (Jas)
Lynch, James Dev.
Lynch, John
Lynch, Michael

Lynch, P.
Lyne, Nealie
Lyne, Dominic

M

Manahan, Jimmy (fleet mechanic)
McCrohan, Dan
McCrohan, Paddy
McCarthy, M.
McCarthy, J.
McCarthy, D.
McEllanory, Ian
Moriarty, Martin
Moriarty, Sandra
Murley, John
Mulloy, Pat
Murphy, C.
Murphy, D.D.
Murphy, Eamon
Murphy, Eddie
Murphy, Frank
Murphy, Jimmy (Jimin)
Murphy, John (Hopper Con)
Murphy, John (Hopper Jack)
Murphy, John (Padgent)
Murphy, Johnny (Blackie)
Murphy, Junior
Murphy, Josie
Murphy, Michael (Siki)
Murphy, M.
Murphy, Nealie
Murphy, Ned (Shore Attendant but sailed with crew on 19 April 1951)
Murphy, Padgent
Murphy, Patrick Siki
Murphy, Patrick
Murphy, Patrick (S)
Murphy, Patsy (Padgent)
Murphy, Paud
Murphy, Paudie
Murphy, Raymond
Murphy, Seamus
Murphy, Sean

Murphy, Seanie (coxswain)
Murphy, Small Paddy
Murphy, Tadgh

N
Naughton, T.

O
O'Connell, Anthony.
O'Connell, Charlie
O'Connell, D.
O'Connell, J.
O'Connell, Jeremiah (coxswain)
O'Connell, Joe
O'Connell, Johnny
O'Connell, Michael (Dore)
O'Connell, Michael (Miko)
O'Connell, Michael
O'Connell, T.
O'Connor, Anthony (bowman)
O'Connor, David
O'Connor, John (Dasher)
O'Connor, John
O'Connor, Michael
O, Connor, Steve
O'Driscoll, D.
O'Driscoll, J.
O'Driscoll, Kieran (honorary secretary) (sailed with crew on 19 April 1951)
O'Donovan, Nealie
O'Leary, Michael (MIKO)
O'Neill, Shane
O'Shea, Con
O'Shea, Johnny (The Rocky) (bowman)
O'Sullivan, Alan
O Sullivan, Gerard
O'Sullivan, Joseph
O Sullivan, H.
O'Sullivan, Paddy (Danny)
O'Sullivan, Michael Sr
O'Sullivan, Michael

Q
Quigley, Andrew
Quigley John
Quigley, Richard

R
Reidy, Gerard
Reidy, John
Ring, Diarmaid
Ring, Kevin
Ring, Padraig
Riordan, P.
Robinson, Richard (Dick)
Ruddock, N.G. (fleet mechanic)

S
Sheehan, John
Sheehan, Tony
Shanahan, John (second coxswain)
Shea, J.
Smyth, Mick
Stewart, T.S. (honorary secretary but went to sea)
Stewart, Pat
Sugrue, Jack (coxswain)
Sugrue, John
Sugrue, John
Sugrue, Paddy
Sullivan, J.

W
Wallace, Syd
Walsh, A.
Walsh, A. (J)
Walsh, Aidan
Walsh, Dermot (coxswain) (Silver Medal)
Walsh, Dermot Jr
Walsh, Dodie
Walsh, Dan
Walsh, Donal
Walsh, John
Walsh, Owen
Walsh, Tony

Watrine, John
Whiz, Bill